D0787860

Sociobiological
Psychiatry

Sociobiological Psychiatry

Normal Behavior and Psychopathology

Brant Wenegrat

Lexington Books

D.C. Heath and Company/Lexington, Massachusetts/Toronto

Library of Congress Cataloging-in-Publication Data

Wenegrat, Brant.
Sociobiological psychiatry : normal behavior and psychopathology
/ Brant Wenegrat.
p.   cm.
ISBN 0–669–21829–4 (alk. paper)
1. Social psychiatry. 2. Sociobiology. I. Title.
RC455.W46   1990
616.89—dc20   89–13963
CIP

Published simultaneously in Canada
Printed in the United States of America
Casebound International Standard Book Number: 0–669–21829–4
Library of Congress Catalog Card Number: 89–13963

The paper used in this publication meets the minimum requirements of
American National Standard for Information Sciences—Permanence of
Paper for Printed Library Materials, ANSI Z39.48–1984. ∞™

The first and last numbers below indicate year and number of printing.

90 91 92 10 9 8 7 6 5 4 3 2 1

Contents

Preface

Fifteen years ago, E.O. Wilson upset a good number of educated citizens by suggesting, in his book *Sociobiology: The New Synthesis,* that human behavior might be understood in evolutionary terms. No one apparently was upset by the bulk of Wilson's book, which described nonhuman behaviors as evolved adaptations, but Wilson's application of a Darwinian framework to human social behaviors stuck in the public craw, so to speak. The controversy resulting from Wilson's book spawned an entire industry. Articles and books were written attacking, defending, or analyzing what was thought to be Wilson's position, and pickets and protests were organized by those more inclined to be physical. In recent years, by contrast, the public controversy over what has come to be called sociobiology has largely disappeared. No one on any side of the issue has changed his or her mind, of course, but the issues have lost their luster in the popular press. There may be an upper limit to public interest in fights between Harvard professors, as the sociobiology debate became, or the public may have realized that more important things were happening. After all, when a significant number of people are living on the streets, as they now do, and when others are dying from a new disease, as they now are, the moral implications of Darwinian theory begin to seem less pressing.

Many people have confused sociobiology with the debate it spawned, so they have been misled in recent years into thinking that sociobiology had waned, or had been a flash in the pan, merely because it no longer attracted public attention. One academic psychologist I know reassured her graduate students that sociobiology had become a thing of the past which, like phrenology, they need not bother to study. To some extent, Wilson's allies have fostered this misimpression. Horrified by the passions they had aroused, many of those who called themselves sociobiologists decided to go underground in the 1980s. They borrowed a leaf from some of the animals they study and camouflaged themselves with new titles, or with old ones, since they were all zoologists, anthropologists, or something else to begin with before they thought of themselves as sociobiologists. The word "sociobiology" dropped out of articles and books, which nonetheless still addressed sociobiological issues, and many people admitted they were unreformed sociobiologists only to their friends, or after they had too much to drink. They spoke about Stephen Jay Gould, the most influential of Wilson's critics, with the same combination of fear and respect old communists I have known reserved for J. Edgar Hoover, and they were only too happy if most people thought they had found new lines of work.

However, in spite of its lower profile in the public press, and the camouflage assumed by some of its advocates, sociobiology is far from becoming extinct. In fact, it is flourishing. Hapless graduate students will have to study it after all. During the last decade, more and more anthropologists, psychologists, zoologists, and others have applied sociobiological models in their discipline and found them to be useful. There is a new emphasis on empirical studies, and a new agreement on the types of data needed. Sociobiological theories have been refined and specified, so their predictions are clearer. Progress is most evident in applying sociobiology to specifically human behaviors. Last year, the Human Behavior and Evolution Society, which has grown more rapidly than its organizers expected, held its first annual meeting at Northwestern University in Evanston, Illinois. Anthropologists, psychologists, psychiatrists, and psychoanalysts, among others, presented papers pertaining to nearly every aspect of human social behavior. Most of the papers presented at this meeting were sociobiological, in the broadest sense.

While sociobiology has been surviving its infancy, psychiatry has been suffering a kind of mid-life crisis. In particular, the remarkable success of the biological revolution in psychiatry has called into question traditional accounts of psychopathology, and especially of the psychological and environmental—in other words, the nonorganic—factors thought to affect mental illness. Nonorganic factors believed to affect mental illness include relationships with parents, siblings, and children, community involvement, job satisfaction, marital status, sexual inhibitions and conflicts, religious feelings, and self-representations, among many others. I will discuss these in this book. Psychiatrists who are aware of the recent advances, but who are sufficiently experienced to know that very few patients can be cured with drugs alone, are especially anxious to find new ways of thinking about nonorganic factors that will be consistent with the biological viewpoint that will dominate future practice. Current ways of thinking about these factors are owed to the social sciences, to behaviorism, and to psychoanalysis, and they cannot be easily integrated with a biological viewpoint. Modern social sciences and behaviorism have, for the most part, specifically eschewed biological thinking. That is why some of Wilson's most fervent critics came from the social sciences. Although psychoanalysis is based in part on the biological thinking of an earlier era, only some of its concepts are consistent with modern biology.

Critics of sociobiology will welcome a "sociobiological psychiatry" with all the enthusiasm they would feel for a measles epidemic. Many people mistakenly think measles has disappeared, along with sociobiology, and would just as soon see the former reappear as the latter. Nonetheless, sociobiological and psychiatric interests currently overlap, providing an opportunity for cross-fertilization and even for development of a sociobiological psychiatry, the form of which is yet to be determined. The fact is that psychological and environmental factors that affect mental illness, and that many psychiatrists would now like to reconceptualize, relate to aspects of social life which sociobiologists consider evolved adaptations. They have already thought about them in biological terms, and the insights they have gained may be useful for psychiatry. In this book, I apply the ideas sociobiologists have had to topics in psychiatry and in clinical practice, in order to show how they how stimulate new ways of thinking about familiar issues.

Acknowledgments

Many people helped me write this book. Adolf Pfefferbaum, Walton T. Roth, and Bert Kopell, among others in the Department of Psychiatry and Behavioral Science at Stanford, provided me with an environment in which I could study and write. Peter Finkelstein encouraged me to continue. The psychiatric residents at Stanford helped me by discussing ideas with me in classes and in clinics. My patients, too, helped me by drawing my attention to important aspects of the problems that bothered them. Stanford University librarians helped me with their unfailing good humor and efficiency. Anne O'Reilly Wenegrat and Jacob O'Reilly Wenegrat gave me their emotional support and were patient with me when I was tired or discouraged.

1
Introduction

My aim in writing this book is to demonstrate that much of the data of modern psychiatry can be effectively organized using relatively few sociobiological models. The data I will organize in this way include clinical and experimental findings on phenomenology, epidemiology, etiology, and treatment of most mental disorders. In the process, I will also paint a picture of normal adaptation with which to compare mental illness. Though my emphasis is mostly behavioral and objective, I hope to lay the groundwork for a new metapsychology applicable to psychodynamic therapy. That is, the organizational scheme outlined in this book can be used to comprehend subjective preoccupations reported by patients with various mental disorders.

Key concepts in psychiatry have been borrowed from or stimulated by models of evolution. The importance Freud ascribed to reproductive, somatic, and aggressive drives, his theory of psychosexual stages, his notions of primal fantasies and organic repression, and his theory of the "primal horde" in *Totem and Taboo* (1913) all follow to some extent from Darwinian models (see Fox, 1980; Sulloway, 1979; also Bock, 1980; Leak and Christopher, 1982). Jung's ideas on archetypes and the collective unconscious are likewise clearly related to the theory of evolution as understood at the time (see Lumsden and Wilson, 1981; Stevens, 1982). Although he opposed "Social Darwinism," Adler's ideas on organ inferiority, compensations, and the compensatory will-to-power express in the psychological realm issues of fitness and adaptation introduced by Darwin into general biology (see Ellenberger, 1970). Most recently, Bowlby (1969, 1973, 1977, 1980) and his followers have reintroduced Darwinian themes into general psychiatry, in the form of "attachment theory." This important body of work is discussed in a later chapter.

Sociobiology is the evolutionary study of animal social life (see, for example, Barash, 1979, 1982; Noonan, 1987; Trivers, 1985; Wilson, 1975). It treats social behavior as an evolved adaptation, akin to bodily form. Sociobiologic models have developed rapidly during the last two decades because of certain advances, methodologic and conceptual, in ethology and biology. In fact, the development has been so rapid that current sociobiological models now have little in common with evolutionary models of social life from twenty or more years ago, which have influenced present-day psychopathological theories. The current models seem to be tailor-made for psychiatry, and a number of authors, myself included, have tried to use them to understand psychiatric disorders (for example, see Badcock, 1986; Buss, 1984; Draper and Harpending, 1988; Gardner, 1982; Glantz and Pearce, 1989; Littlefield and Rushton, 1986; McGuire and Essock-Vitale, 1981; McGuire and Fairbanks, 1977; McGuire, et al., 1981; Nesse, 1984; Price, 1967, 1969, 1972; Price and Sloman, 1984; Slavin, 1985; Slavin and Kriegman, 1988; Sloman, 1981, 1983; Sloman, et al., 1979; Wenegrat, 1984). I and others believe that sociobiology now offers psychiatry an encompassing basic science, akin to what quantum physics offers modern chemistry.

In response to my previous effort, a number of colleagues have told me, in more or less gentle terms, that I might have spared the trouble, that psychiatry needs no "encompassing basic science," much less one tainted by the hint of political scandal (see below). Clinical practice will always reside in the ingenious application of specific facts—biologic, cultural, and personal—regardless of whether these facts form a coherent whole from some single vantage point. I have been told that as long as we have useful facts, and continue to gather new ones, an encompassing viewpoint like the one I aimed to demonstrate is just excess baggage.

I think that this critique takes an excessively narrow view of the psychiatric endeavor. First, even psychiatrists wholly occupied with clinical work appreciate some coherence in the various facts they try to employ. Cognitive psychologists find that people try to fit facts and ideas together in an automatic and somewhat compulsive manner. When they succeed, they feel some kind of pleasure. This, presumably, is one reason modern physicists keep trying to find a "unified field theory," rather than being content with the elegant but disunited field theories they currently have in hand. I assume that psychiatrists are really no different. If achieving some coherence among seemingly disparate facts and ideas provides some pleasure to them, I think this effort is justified.

Among the various facts and ideas in modern psychiatry, those pertaining to diagnosis seem especially in need of coherence. Diagnosis is the foundation for any clinical science. Yet the present diagnostic system in psychiatry is based on a potpourri of unrelated concepts. This is especially true for personality problems (see, for example, Docherty, et al., 1986; Frances and Widiger, 1986; Hirschfeld, 1986; Siever and Klar, 1986). Although individual diagnoses are statistically reliable, there is no encompassing scheme that shows their interrelations. By contrast, today's medical diagnosticians employ a coherent system. Their diagnoses refer to specific organs or systems. They diagnose disorders of the heart, lung, or immune system, to take a few examples. Anatomy and physiology provide an encompassing framework with a place for each disorder. A major aim of this book is to reference behavioral diagnoses to sociobiological concepts. Specifically I will show that certain strategies described by sociobiologists provide an encompassing framework for behavioral diagnoses. These strategies offer psychiatry what organs and functional systems provide for general medicine.

Second, psychiatrists pursue research. And research is mostly guided by the way facts seem to cohere, by hypothetical models. For example, the reason we know much at all about schizophrenic genetics is that facts concerning the illness—including its aggregation in families and amelioration by biologic treatments—could be made to cohere with each other by presuming genetic causes. In other words, facts about schizophrenia could be assimilated to a preexisting "genetic disorder" model derived from other sources. This model prompted studies that proved highly productive. More recently, a hypothetical model concerning the importance of early attachment has stimulated research on child-mother relationships. If the data of modern psychiatry cohere in light of sociobiologic models, those models might guide the direction of future research. For the most part research is guided by models that are more mechanistic than sociobiological models tend to be. Yet I think it safe to say that sociobiological models applied to psychiatric data do point out avenues of special theoretical interest, and that some researchers may want to pursue those leads.

Finally, unless we put our heads in the sand, we psychiatrists and other mental health professionals will sooner or later encounter sociobiological ideas. We will sooner or later use them to rethink psychopathology. We may as well do so now. For sociobiology, in effect, is on psychiatry's home ground: the biology of the mind. Sociobiological concepts—like psychoanalytic ones eighty years ago—produce a new view of the mind in the broadest possible sense. And though these concepts come from an area of biology unfamiliar to us and to other physicians, the view they engender is as biological as one based on neuroanatomy. It is only more abstract.

This book follows a very simple plan. Chapter 2 describes a model of human social behavior based on Darwinian theory and sociobiological concepts. This model emphasizes certain behavior patterns, which I will call here "innately probable strategies." In my previous work I called these "genetically transmitted strategies." However, regardless of the precautions I took, certain terms in that work involving the word "genetic" led to some confusion. I have therefore tried to avoid them here. Innately probable strategies are the building blocks of normal human social life.

Chapters 3 and 4 describe particular innately probable strategies. Strategies are grouped together according to whether they are concerned with childlike aid–seeking, relationships with social groups, or adult competition. Insofar as they are known, factors are discussed that predispose persons to adhere to particular strategies.

In chapters 3 and 4, I will try to show that psychiatric syndromes are aberrant manifestations of innately probable strategies. I will try to specify what has gone wrong with a particular strategy to produce a particular syndrome. All sorts of observations— concerning phenomenology, etiology, epidemiology, treatment, and prognosis of particular syndromes—will be reexamined for their strategic meaning.

Chapter 5 discusses pathogenetic factors producing mental disorders and factors that might be altered in the course of treatment. In chapter 5 I will try to show how sociobiological models affect clinical thinking. Chapter 5 is brief; it offers an introduction to issues of clinical practice which, thoroughly discussed, would comprise a separate volume.

Various authors allege that sociobiological ideas justify repression, racism, gender discrimination, and a Hobbesian view of society (for examples, see Caplan, 1978; Lewontin, et al., 1984; Montagu, 1980; Sahlins, 1976). The moral and political issues raised by these and other authors have been thoughtfully discussed by biologists, anthropologists, ethicists, and philosophers (see, for example, Alexander, 1979; Breuer, 1982; Caplan, 1978; Gruter and Bohannan, 1983; Ingold, 1986; Lopreato, 1984; Maxwell, 1984; Ruse, 1987; Silverman, 1987; Stent, 1978a; Wilson, 1978a). In my opinion, all but one of the political and moral objections to sociobiological concepts have been well refuted, and require no further attention here. The single exception, the charge that sociobiology is inherently antifeminist, is discussed below.

Many authors attacking sociobiological concepts have actually misunderstood them in elementary ways. They have confused sociobiology with simple genetic determinism or have reified "inclusive fitness." Readers interested in the first issue are referred to MacDonald (1988a), who explained how theories of genetic determinism differ from sociobiological theories, and to Fuller (1987) who explained the limitations of genetic determinism, even in the field of behavior genetics, which tries to directly measure it. Inclusive fitness is defined in chapter 2. Certain writers, who are more propagandists than scholars, create straw creatures they call sociobiology, which they then show are socially irresponsible. Readers exposed to these caricatures may be surprised by the real thing. Sociobiological ideas— and the views they engender—are elegant and subtle. I have yet to see these qualities conveyed in the popular press, which has provided a forum for attacks on the field.

Sociobiological theories concern "human nature." The sociobiological view is that human nature can be defined, if only in probabilistic, somewhat contingent terms. Belief in the reality of human nature, and consequently in the reality of human needs and values independent of particular social arrangements, is an important safeguard to individual freedom, at least if that nature is not misconstrued so as to promote or excuse evil (see, for example, Chomsky, 1975; Silverman, 1987; Tiger, 1979; Wilson, 1978b). It is not coincidental that psychological "experts"—trained in a theoretical system that denies human nature except as a social construction—have helped to suppress dissent in the Soviet Union (see Fromm, 1961). So–called tabula rasa theories popular among Western academic and clinical psychologists have eroded distinctions previously drawn between social convention and moral conduct (Turiel, 1978; see also Wolff, 1978). The result has been that Western psychological theorists, too, endorse regnant social norms while ignoring moral concerns (see also Wallach and Wallach, 1983). In the process they lend themselves to support of the status quo, and they undermine the philosophy on which our political system is necessarily based.

Claims that sociobiology is antifeminist have been dealt with less adequately than other political issues. Feminists, of course, are sensitive to the ways in which evolutionary theories have been used to suppress women's aspirations (see, Dijkstra, 1986), and therefore they are biased against sociobiology, which has assumed the Darwinian mantle. But there are at least two issues raised by sociobiology that might disturb them, even if women had not been treated poorly in the past by evolutionary theories. First, sociobiological models of male reproductive strategies seem to imply that men see women as reproductive machines, valued for their wombs but otherwise quite dispensable. This is in spite of the fact that, at least at their best, men seem to be capable of appreciating women for all the same reasons they appreciate men. Second, sociobiological models of female reproductive strategies seem to imply that women wish to depend on wealthy and powerful men, rather than to support themselves. This is in spite of the fact that throughout human history, and, as far as we can tell, in prehistoric times, women have worked as hard to support men and their families as men have worked to support women (see Anderson and Zinsser, 1988). Wealthy and powerful women have been as much sought by men as wealthy and powerful men have been sought by women.

I think it is correct to say that sociobiological theories impose no particular limits on the types of interests men may take in women, in addition to those which are sexual. If in some current societies men see women as purely sexual objects, rather than as people, this is the result of cultural constraints on the types of relationships men and women may cultivate, rather than of biology. Sociobiological models do predict that in societies where men control resources needed for rearing children, women will try to obtain guarantees of aid from men before reproducing. To do otherwise would be foolish, regardless of one's theoretical framework. Also, in these societies, men will compete with each other to control useful resources as a means of obtaining women. But there is nothing in sociobiology that implies that depending on powerful men is desirable to women. In fact, women should prefer to be powerful in their own right and to be independent of men. In chapter 4, I mention alternative sexual strategies that women might pursue if they controlled resources needed for rearing children.

When due regard is paid to the highly contingent nature of reproductive strategies, which are nonetheless "innately probable" in the sense I will describe, I think that sociobiological models lead to a picture of male-female relationships somewhat like Frederick Engels's. Engels (1972) argued that male control of productive resources—achieved by force—led to subjugation of women in historical times. Engels called this process the "defeat of the female sex." According to Engels, emancipation of women can only be accomplished if they regain full partnership in control of productive resources. Leacock (1972) discussed Engels's thesis in light of current knowledge of early cultural history, and Hrdy (1981) briefly reviewed it in light of primate data. Unfortunately, a full discussion of Engels's thesis in sociobiological terms in a daunting project that has yet to be tackled.

The importance of coming to grips with the feminist issue before it further poisons the atmosphere around sociobiology is shown by a recent book, addressed to psychotherapists (Glantz and Pearce, 1989). The authors of this book describe what they believe are evolved sex roles, the implication being that these are more compatible with mental health than alternative roles. The authors of this book pay insufficient attention to whether the roles they identify really serve fitness interests in all societies, or whether they serve the interests of both sexes. They fail to consider that these roles may be inherently conflict-ridden and cause dissatisfaction for men, women, or both. This is because their argument suffers from the intrusion of "group-selectionist" thinking (see chapter 3), which sociobiologists try to avoid. One commentator quoted on the book jacket predicted that feminists would be angered by the authors' position! If so, it will only do further damage to the reputation of sociobiology and slow the diffusion of sociobiological concepts into other fields.

Many of the ideas discussed in this book are speculative. Taken as a whole, this book is a speculation: that sociobiological models can organize the data of modern psychiatry. Speculation on this scale is out of fashion in psychiatry which has tried to restrict itself to discovering new facts. Yet, psychiatry needs more speculation, although it may prove wrong, as to how facts fit together. Our facts today are like loose bricks. The mortar to make something with them will be mixed from speculations that survive the test of time.

2
Basic Concepts

The purpose of this study is to show that innately probable strategies described by sociobiologists account for the major facets of normal human behavior and provide a heuristic framework for interpreting psychopathology. In this chapter, I will describe criteria for identifying innately probable strategies. But first, the reader must be familiar with "inclusive fitness." Inclusive fitness is a vital concept for sociobiological models.

Inclusive Fitness

Darwin (1859) hypothesized that living species are mutable. Better adapted forms replace the less adapted. In this century, after the rediscovery of Mendelian genetics, Darwin's hypothesis was refined. The result is called "neo-Darwinism" (see Dobzhansky, 1951; Mayr, 1963; Simpson, 1953a). Here is the neo-Darwinian model, in highly simplified form: Various processes (for example, mutation, recombination) introduce genetic variation into a breeding population. Due to this variation, members of the population differ in ways that affect their reproductive success. Reproductive success is the number of offspring produced that survive to reproductive age. Because progeny carry parental genes, more successful variants become more and more common with each generation. The population slowly changes. If it is isolated, the population may change so much that its members can no longer breed with their ancestral forms. New species are formed this way.

The neo-Darwinian model has been challenged in recent years by the "neutral theory," the theory of "punctuated equilibrium," and

evidence of acquired inheritable characteristics. These are highly
technical topics beyond the scope of this study. Readers are referred
to Maynard Smith's (1982c) anthology on these issues.

In spite of its overall success, the neo-Darwinian model failed to
explain "altruistic" behaviors. In neo-Darwinian terms, altruistic
behaviors are actions that decrease the actor's expected reproductive
success in order to increase the expected reproductive success of
another individual (see Bertram, 1982). "Expected" is intended here
in a purely statistical sense, since the actual consequence of an act
is largely a matter of chance. For example, if an altruist, A, leaves a
safe haven to save a beneficiary, B, who is not A's progeny, from a
predator, A's expected reproductive success will decrease as a result
of the risk he or she incurs and B's will increase as the result of
the greater chance of escape he or she gains. Altruistic behaviors
are essential to social species, and especially to higher primates and
humans.

Neo-Darwinian "altruism" is only partly related to "altruism" in
its common usage. In particular, neo-Darwinian altruism implies no
intention to render aid, only that aid is actually rendered (Stent,
1978b).

Hamilton (1964) provided the key suggestion as to how neo-
Darwinism might be modified to account for altruistic behaviors.
This suggestion had been foreseen by Fisher (1930) and Haldane
(1932), founders of neo-Darwinism, but never fully integrated into
the neo-Darwinian model. Relatives other than parents and offspring
carry copies of the same ancestral genes. The degree of genetic
kinship between any two individuals A and B can be expressed as
a coefficient, ranging from 0, for totally unrelated individuals, to 1,
for identical twins. This coefficient is calculated from elementary
genetic information (see, for example, Stern, 1960). If A and B are
related by r, where r is a coefficient, then r is also the chance that
B will carry a copy of a given autosomal ancestral gene inherited by
A. A and B can be interchanged here, the relationship being symmet-
rical. The situation is somewhat more complicated for genes on the
X and Y chromosomes. In what follows, it should be understood
that the models refer to autosomal genes. Hamilton pointed out that
an individual's Darwinian fitness—that is, the number of copies of
his or her genes that result from that individual's activity—is incom-

pletely measured by reproductive success. Reproductive success accounts for copies carried by progeny but not for copies carried by relatives whose survival to reproductive age might be influenced by the individual in question. In other words, if we want to measure an individual's influence on the propagation of his or her genes, we have to account for how that individual affects his relatives who carry copies of those genes, and not merely for progeny. Hamilton called the wider measure "inclusive fitness." The term speaks for itself.

I will give two examples to illustrate how inclusive fitness is calculated: An individual, A, has eight progeny who reach reproductive age. A belongs to a solitary-living mammalian species; his activity has no effect on his other kin. The coefficient of relatedness between parent and offspring is 0.5; consequently, there is a 50 percent chance that a given gene carried by A is carried by each of his progeny. Therefore, A's activity is expected, in a statistical sense, to produce four copies (8 times 0.5) of any of A's genes. A's inclusive fitness is four. The units are understood to be copies of A's genes. A's inclusive fitness equals his reproductive success. Another individual, B, has four progeny who reach reproductive age. B belongs to a social mammalian species; his activity has an effect on his genetic kin. Specifically, protection he gives to four younger full siblings permits each to reach reproductive age, which they would not have reached without B's help. The coefficient of relatedness between full siblings is 0.5; consequently, there is a 50 percent chance that a given ancestral gene carried by B is carried by each of his siblings. B's inclusive fitness is also four. Half of these (4 times 0.5) are accounted for by B's reproductive success. Half (4 times 0.5) are accounted for by his aid to his siblings, which allowed them to reach reproductive age.

If we studied A and B purely in terms of reproductive success, we would have erroneously concluded that A is better adapted than B.

If we change the neo-Darwinian model so that inclusive fitness takes the place of reproductive success, it becomes clear how altruistic behaviors involving kin can evolve. Recall that these behaviors reduce the actor's reproductive success, and so could not be accounted for by the original model. In terms of the new model: If the actor's decreased reproductive success is compensated for by enhanced reproductive success of kin carrying the same ancestral genes, then the action in question will not be maladaptive, in the sense of reducing fitness. If the benefits to kin—depreciated according to their degree of relatedness—exceed the loss to the actor, the action in question will be favored by selection.

In general, if C (for Cost) is the loss of reproductive potential incurred by an altruist, B is the expected benefit in reproductive potential accruing to the recipient, and r is the degree of genetic relatedness between altruist and recipient, then altruistic acts satisfying the relation:

$$rB > C \qquad\qquad (2.1)$$

will increase inclusive fitness. Recall that r varies between zero and one. Acts like these are adaptive. Altruistic acts failing to satisfy relation (2.1) will be maladaptive, depending upon the degree to which C exceeds rB.

Behaviors that decrease reproductive success but increase inclusive fitness because of their effects on genetic kin are said to benefit from positive "kin selection." This is a way of saying that natural selection proceeds in this case by way of enhanced reproduction of kin.

The conditions described in equation (2.1) dictate a "strategy" for advantageous altruism: "Perform altruistic acts that satisfy this equation." Adherence to this strategy will enhance inclusive fitness in comparison with alternative strategies: indiscriminate altruism without regard for equation (2.1) or indiscriminate refusal to be altruistic at all. In this way, adherence to a strategy can be said to confer inclusive fitness benefits, or penalties, should the strategy be inferior. The inclusive fitness effect of a particular strategy is always a relative matter that depends upon the alternatives. In what follows, I will discuss inclusive fitness mainly in terms of strategies.

When sociobiologists say that individuals adhere to particular strategies, they do not mean to imply that these individuals have any awareness whatsoever of inclusive fitness effects. Authors unfamiliar with sociobiology sometimes claim that individuals try to "maximize" their inclusive fitness, or that they calculate the inclusive fitness consequences of particular actions. Nothing could be more misleading. According to sociobiologists, humans and other animals have evolved dispositional factors and mental processes (see below) that produce adherence to strategies that confer selective advantages. The inclusive fitness advantages and the strategies per se are wholly outside awareness and have no motivational role.

Genes are also said to confer inclusive fitness, or to detract from it. The rationale for this is as follows: In calculating an individual's inclusive fitness, we count the number of gene copies expected to result from the varied strategies to which he or she adheres. Insofar as carrying a certain gene alters the probability of adherence to certain strategies, that gene will alter the inclusive fitness of its carriers. The incremental inclusive fitness change experienced by carriers is the inclusive fitness detracted or conferred by the gene.

Imagine, for example, that individual A above heterozygously carried a gene that made him mate more frequently, producing more than eight progeny. In a later chapter, I will show how mating efforts are described in strategic terms. His inclusive fitness (and reproductive success) might be increased by this gene, according to the number of additional progeny he produced. A's incremental fitness gain as the result of this gene is said to be conferred by the gene. This is a relative number; the baseline inclusive fitness from which incremental changes are calculated depends upon alternative genes that A might otherwise carry. Also, a given gene may have differing fitness effects in the presence of differing genes at other genetic loci, or when present in homozygous form.

Genes detract from inclusive fitness if they decrease fitness in comparison with the alternatives. Imagine, for example, that individual B above heterozygously carried a gene that somehow diminished his desire to help his siblings, so that he aided only two of them, instead of four as he would have if he carried the usual gene. In strategic terminology, the gene would have the effect of making B's adherence to the strategy in equation (2.1) rather more haphazard. B's inclusive fitness would then be three, instead of four. As before, two of these units are gained through reproductive success; only one unit is gained now from aid given to kin. In comparison with the alternative gene that B was presumed to carry, the new gene can be said to detract one unit from inclusive fitness.

Universal and Evolutionarily Stable Strategies

A "universal" human strategy is one that is ubiquitous in every human society. If there are societies in which it is not in evidence, there should be clearly comprehensible reasons for its apparent absence. For example, if a society is such that persons living in it are never exposed to the situation to which the strategy applies, then the strategy could not be expected to be very much in evidence. To return to equation (2.1), if there were a society in which no one lived near anyone they considered even remotest kin (an impossible situation for reasons discussed in a later chapter), then kin-altruistic acts specified by equation (2.1) would not be expected to occur. The strategy embodied in equation (2.1) would be a moot point. Individuals from past societies, insofar as their behavior can be reconstructed, should also have adhered to universal strategies, as may some nonhuman primates. Chimpanzees, who are the non-human primates genetically closest to human beings, and baboons, who occupy an ecological niche similar to that occupied by early hominids, will be of special interest in this regard.

Universality alone does not prove that a strategy is biologically determined, except in a trivial sense. For example, people every-where work—either growing and producing or gathering what they need—and it might be said that the disposition to work is inherent in human biology. But while it is perfectly true that human biology dictates certain needs that can only be met by the "strategy" of work-ing, a biologic account of work would be a pointless exercise. The more interesting factors affecting work are environmental ones: some environments make it easier to meet biologic needs. And the most interesting factors are cultural: technology, systems of economic organization, and creation of superfluous needs determine the nature and tempo of work as well as its distribution.

Evolutionarily stable strategies are superior, in inclusive fitness terms, to alternative strategies that might threaten to take their place (Davies, 1982; Maynard Smith, 1976, 1982b). Consequently, genes promoting adherence to evolutionarily stable strategies cannot be replaced by genes promoting adherence to alternative strategies, because the latter will detract from inclusive fitness. For example, the kin-altruistic strategy embodied in equation (2.1) will always be more advantageous than its two alternatives: indiscriminate altruism without regard for cost, kinship, and benefit, or indiscriminate failure to aid anyone at all. Genes that promote indiscriminate altruism or indiscriminate failure to help will detract from inclusive fitness in comparison with genes that promote adherence to altruism as defined by equation (2.1). Genes promoting indiscriminate altruism or indiscriminate failure to help would fail to spread, or even to hold their own, in competition with genes promoting kin-altruism.

The kin-altruistic strategy embodied in equation (2.1) is evolutionarily stable regardless of its frequency in a given population. An individual kin altruist will maximize his inclusive fitness no matter how others behave with respect to their own kin. However, this is an exception. In general, strategies become evolutionarily stable only when they are used by nearly all individuals in a given population. There is typically a critical (majority) proportion of the population, such that evolutionary stability develops only when the number of individuals using the strategy exceeds that proportion. When the proportion is reached, individuals adhering to "deviant" strategies will suffer diminished inclusive fitness in comparison with the majority. In other cases, a combination of strategies can be evolutionarily stable; if mixed in the right proportions, two or more strategies can effectively penalize deviant alternatives. In such cases, single individuals may use different component strategies with particular frequencies, or a particular proportion of the population may use one strategy, while the remainder use another. Examples of each possibility are cited in later chapters.

I will illustrate here the simplest case, in which evolutionary stability depends upon nearly unanimous use of a strategy in a population. Suppose the members of an isolated religious commune decided for theologic reasons to institute the following program: No communard is permitted to provide any aid whatsoever to a first-degree relative, regardless of age. First-degree relatives include parents, children, or siblings. These are the very persons equation (2.1) predicts would receive the most aid. But religion has been known to oppose biologic preference, so the example here, while improbable, isn't quite inconceivable. Children, of course, would have to be raised by foster parents, or by aunts, uncles, or cousins. In order to enforce this prohibition, members of the commune agree to execute those who receive forbidden aid.

The program dictates a strategy: to avoid at least direct aid to first degree kin. If nearly everyone in the group adheres to and enforces this strategy and if there is insufficient privacy in the group to allow secret aid, then the strategy is evolutionarily stable against the social deviant who insists on aiding first degree kin. An individual who deviated from the consensual strategy by directly aiding first degree kin would condemn his own closest relatives and thereby decrease his inclusive fitness.

Like universality, evolutionary stability alone does not prove that a strategy has biological causes. The above example, in which theology dictates a hypothetical strategy, should make that clear. The strategy is no less stable because of its cultural origin.

Throughout this book, I will use the initials "ESS" to refer to an evolutionarily stable strategy. In doing so I am following common practice.

Innately probable strategies are strategies which result nontrivially from gene activity. Presumably, genes can promote behavioral dispositions which increase the probability of adherence to particular strategies, given certain environmental conditions. Universal ESS's can be assumed to be innately probable strategies.

Consider again the hypothetical religious community described above. If it remained isolated for many generations, and if no political or theologic upheavals disrupted the consensual ban on aiding close kin, then the evolutionary stability of the strategy dictated by the group would gradually produce individuals more amenable to it. Because attempts to aid close kin would usually wind up killing them, genes that predisposed toward undisguised adherence to the strategy of equation (2.1) would gradually disappear from the community's gene pool. Instead of conferring added inclusive fitness, as they do in normal circumstances, in the setting of this particular group they would decrease inclusive fitness until they disappeared. Were ties reestablished with members of other groups, the lack of apparent familial feeling in members of the formerly isolated community would no doubt surprise their new acquaintances. The degree to which feelings had atrophied would depend on the duration of isolation, the group's ability to detect and punish kin altruism, the extent to which genetic effects contribute to these feelings, and the degree of genetic diversity present in the group when altruism was first proscribed.

In other words, if an ESS is ubiquitous and long-standing, so that selective pressures against alternative strategies are maintained for extremely long periods of time, then those selective pressures will eventually fix the ESS in the community gene pool. This will occur through selection against genetically caused predispositions that intrude on adherence to the ESS; what will be left are the genes and predispositions that promote adherence instead. This will occur regardless of how the ESS is initially spread. As the example above shows, even a culturally determined ESS will, given adequate time, eliminate competing dispositions dependent on gene activity. If an ESS is universal within a social group, and has been universal for a long enough time, then nature—represented by genetically mediated dispositional factors (of the types discussed below)—must not only acquiesce but collude in its propagation.

I am assuming, of course, that there actually are dispositional factors dependent on gene activity that affect the chance of adherence to particular ESS's. If no such factors existed, the longest-standing ESS could never be fixed in the gene pool in the sense described above. An ESS, of course, is always a social strategy. By definition an ESS impinges on other persons. There is now a body of evidence that human social interactions do depend on innate dispositional factors of a type that can affect the chance of adherence to ESS's. Because of the theoretical importance of this point, I will briefly review this evidence in the following section.

This argument, to the effect that adherence to a universal ESS must be innately probable, is similar in form to one made by the early evolutionary theorist James Mark Baldwin (1896). Baldwin was trying to show that learned adaptations can become genetically fixed through purely Darwinian processes. According to Baldwin, learned behavioral adaptations lead to selective pressures in favor of modifications—mental and anatomic—that promote their effective performance (see also Chisholm, 1988; Richards, 1987). Mayr (1963) and Simpson (1953b) reviewed certain problems with the process Baldwin hypothesized. The so-called Baldwin Effect is similar to a process Waddington (1953a, 1953b) later named "genetic assimilation." Waddington showed that genetic assimilation occurs in animal models. There is also a connection between the Baldwin Effect and Piagetian theories of cognitive development (see Cahan, 1984; Piaget, 1978).

Innate Dispositions Affecting Social Strategies

Several types of dispositions—perceptual, cognitive, affective and motivational, communicative and gestural, and motorically stereotyped—direct the course of social life into more probable channels. I will provide examples of these and show that they are innate. The discussion here is necessarily brief. Readers wishing to learn more are referred to the studies cited below.

Within the first hours of life perceptual dispositions appear which affect later social relations. These dispositions cannot be produced by learning and so must be somehow preprogrammed in the nervous system. The nervous system, of course, is formed through expression of genes. In particular, the neonate shows a striking preference for viewing the human face (Fantz, 1963; Spitz, 1965), and a marked attentiveness to the sound of the human voice (Friedlander, 1970). Neonates apparently distinguish the sound of their mother's voice from that of other women (DeCasper and Fifer, 1980). Neonates' ability to recognize a particular voice is no doubt due to hearing it during intrauterine life, but it does show a disposition to make perceptual distinctions of great social importance appearing very early on. Other stimulus preferences in newborn humans and animals have been extensively studied and are also vital to forming early social relations (see, for example, MacFarlane, 1975; Rosenblatt, 1976; Russell, 1976; Sherrod, 1981).

Very young infants perceptually "quantize" speech sounds into categorical phonemes used in human languages (Eimas, 1985; Eimas, et al., 1971). This perceptual disposition occurs too early to be accounted for by exposure to speech. Furthermore, some of the categorical distinctions made by infants may not even be found in the language they later learn and so will be lost through disuse. Phonemic perceptual processes are essential to language acquisition and depend on specialized cortical sites (Liberman, 1979; Luria, 1981; Marler, 1979; Ploog, 1979).

Very early in life, infants can discriminate certain facial expressions (Field, et al., 1982). Infants can also remember particular facial features following brief exposures (Fagan, 1973, 1976). Expression and facial perception are obviously important to maintaining social relations. Facial recognition depends upon cortical loci separate from those responsible for general pattern perception (Geshwind, 1979).

As the infant matures, he or she becomes sensitive to facial, vocal, and motor cues shown by caretaking figures. Stern (1985) has summarized data showing how thoroughly "tuned in" infants are to their mothers (and vice versa, of course). The infants' sensitivity can hardly be accounted for by previous learning contingencies; instead it must reflect an innate attentiveness to maternal behavior. Through its responsiveness, the infant strengthens the bond on which its survival depends.

Adult perceptual dispositions are potentially modified by environmental and cultural factors. Nonetheless, adults everywhere are attuned to perceive certain gestalts with predictable social meanings (cf. Robinson, 1979, on "constructive realism"). Configurations of facial movements, postures, and rhythmic patterns of limb movement are perceived as wholes indicative of affective states (see Buck, 1984; Zivin, 1985). Humans are also attuned to perceive universal dominance signs, or signs of potential submissiveness (see Ellyson and Dovidio, 1985). That perceptual dispositions related to affect and dominance are in fact innate is illustrated by comparing them with perceptual dispositions governing conversation. Conversational gestures are perceived quite differently in different cultures (Ekman, 1979). Also, right hemisphere lesions can impair perception of affect in other persons' speech, without affecting perception of its informational content (Cassem, 1988; Ross and Rush, 1981).

Many universal cognitive dispositions are discussed in later chapters. For example, in a later chapter I will argue that humans everywhere tend to categorize other persons according to their membership in exclusive in-groups, and to take this categorization into greater account than more personal features in deciding upon their attitude toward them. In the same chapter, I will attempt to show that individuals everywhere adopt the cognitions of their in-group, even if that requires ignoring contradictory evidence. Both of these dispositions, and many others, are plausibly dependent upon innate processes. I will even go so far as to argue that we now know something about the neurochemistry of consensual cognitive dispositions.

Jungian archetypes are obviously relevant here. Archetypes,

according to Jung (1919), are inherited dispositions toward species-typical subjective experiences, including cognitive ones. In response to certain events, these dispositions might produce cognitions in part determined by evolution. The archetypes, according to Jung (1919), force human "perception and apprehension into specifically human patterns." The in-group, out-group distinction described in the previous paragraph is clearly archetypal, in this most elementary sense. Numerous other examples like it are found in following chapters. Jungian analysts have tried to show cross-cultural formal themes in works of art and fantasy (see, for example, Neumann 1955). If nothing else these suggest that themes and ideas that occur to people in different cultures are as like each other in form as the actual lives they lead. Evidence of familial obsessional and phobic ideas (Epstein, 1980) and dream content (Epstein and Collie, 1976) makes it appear more plausible that at least some of these themes and ideas emerge because of genes. Stevens (1982) discussed the concept of archetype in ethologic terms, and Lumsden and Wilson (1981) discussed "innate knowledge structures." I discussed archetypes in my earlier work on religious beliefs (Wenegrat 1990).

Naive learning theory treats the nervous system as a *tabula rasa* sensitive to contingencies (see Robinson, 1979). This type of theory seems to preclude a role for innate cognitions. Innate cognitions can play a role in structuring mental activity only insofar as the nervous system is not a *tabula rasa* and resists the effects of contingencies. The nervous system, in fact, is not a *tabula rasa*. For instance, avoidance responses to stimuli associated with naturally occurring dangers, especially predators, cannot be accounted for by previous learning contingencies. Instead, they are innate. Marks (1987) reviewed this data in his study of human phobias. Also, though associations likely to have been important in nature can be learned quite readily, certain others cannot be learned at all (for studies on eating aversions, see Garcia and Koelling, 1966; Garcia, et al., 1972; Rozin and Kalat, 1971; for an overview, see Hinde and Stevenson-Hinde, 1973). In later chapters, I will present evidence that certain associations advantageous in social life in varying cultural settings are quite readily learned, while other associations, which might decrease inclusive fitness, are not learned at all. The most striking example of this is in the sexual realm, in gender-related differences in fetishistic behavior.

Another type of innate cognitive disposition, less obvious than universal categories, archetypes, or constraints on associational learning, is the tendency to think in social terms in the first place. Studies of primitive societies suggest that for hundreds of thousands of years the bulk of selective pressures shaping human intellect was due to social, rather than to natural, exigencies (see chapter 5). That is, skillful performance of social roles and adherence to social strategies have been more important in determining inclusive fitness than problem solving with respect to the natural world. Insofar as selective pressures shaping human cognition have come from the social arena, human intellect has evolved to perform specific functions—those required by the ESS's described in later chapters—and not to solve problems chosen at random. Human cognition, in effect, is "dedicated" to social games, embodied in ESS's. It is more akin to an electronic chess player than to a general purpose computer.

Dedicated computers are designed to perform particular tasks with maximal efficiency, or to be maximally efficient with given types of tasks. When performing other tasks, their speed may be slowed by their suboptimal design. General purpose computers, by contrast, are designed to perform tasks of several types with more or less equal efficiency. Their designs are compromises between the requirements for efficient operation with several types of programs. To say that human cognition is dedicated to social games—the ESS's described in later chapters—is to say that social analyses, needed to support ESS's, are what the human mind does best. Human cognitive skills may be put to any use, but not with the same efficiency.

The social analyses needed for skillful adherence to various ESS's will become more obvious in later chapters. Briefly, with an eye on their cultural norms, humans must be able to categorize others as reliable or not, to judge power relationships dependent on social-political networks and not on physical size, to surmise hidden actors and potentially hidden intentions behind complex events, to trace kinship relations, to imitate authority figures, to see their own actions from the point of view of others and to calculate the responses these others will likely make, and to creatively compromise when interests are in conflict.

In a previous work, I argued that humans address most problems by performing the social analyses which come most easily to them (Wenegrat, 1990). The implications of this view are cited in chapter 5.

In recent years, cognitions and affects have been found to be linked to each other, so that to discuss one is necessarily to discuss the other (cf. Buck, 1976, 1984; Manstead and Wagner, 1981; Schachter, 1964; Schachter and Singer, 1962). Nonetheless, evolutionary theorists in general and sociobiologists in particular have stressed the role of emotion, as opposed to cognition, in controlling contingent behaviors (see, for example, Crawford, 1987; MacDonald, 1988b; Kellerman, 1980; Weinrich, 1980). Affective responses determining social behaviors are now known to be governed in part by nervous structures that are the products of genes (for an overview, see Berger and Brodie, 1986; Gerner and Bunney, 1986; Kaplan and Sadock, 1985; Lishman, 1987). For example, lesions or drugs affecting the limbic system can produce or alleviate depression, euphoria, anxiety, or anger. Lesion or drug-induced mood alterations have far-reaching social effects. As one might expect in light of this type of data, genetic studies have shown that mood disorders are heritable (see chapter 3).

There are many innate motoric patterns with wide-ranging social effects. In animals, for example, tendencies to assume sexual postures are apparently determined by prenatal androgen levels, that affect the developing brain (see chapter 4). These levels in turn are mostly determined by a genetic factor, the presence or absence of the male chromosome. Stereotyped motor patterns are evident in the maternal-child relationship, in which they play an important role (see chapter 3). Emotional gestures are essential to social relations in higher primate species (see Buck, 1984); for the most part they are innate. They appear early in the neonatal period (Izard, 1978; Trevarthen, 1979), develop without the aid of visual experience (Eibl-Eibesfeldt, 1973), and universally signify specific affective states (Ekman, 1979). Similar gestures signify social status and dominance (see Harper, 1985; Keating, 1985; Patterson, 1985). Innate gestures indicative of submission may be important in certain mental disorders (chapter 4).

Consistent with the notion that genes affect nonverbal communication, identical twins raised with little or no contact nonetheless share similar facial expressions, postural habits, and gestures (Farber, 1981).

To illustrate how innate dispositions might affect social behavior patterns, I will return here to the strategy embodied in equation (2.1) and to its counterpart in the hypothetical commune. Adherence to the strategy embodied in equation (2.1) necessitates directing aid toward close kin, with whom the coefficient of relationship, r, is largest. For parents, sons and daughters are close kin who, especially when young, can be expected to benefit greatly from acts performed at relatively little cost. This matter is discussed further in the following chapter. Consequently, parents—and for other reasons explained later, especially mothers—should be anxious to help their children survive their early years. Except in unusual cases, this is in fact the general rule.

Numerous processes dependent upon gene action enhance the concern parents feel for children, and consequently the likelihood that they will offer them aid. To cite just one example, maternal affection for the newborn, as well as caretaking behavior, is stimulated greatly by contact with the newborn shortly after birth (see Ali and Lowry, 1981; Carlsson, et al., 1978; DeChateau and Wiberg, 1977a, 1977b; Hales, et al., 1977; Klaus, et al., 1972; O'Connor, et al., 1977; Trowell, 1982). It seems very likely that neuroendocrine changes at the time of delivery somehow "prime" the mother to develop affective bonds. Maternal endocrine changes depend on genetic activity.

In the hypothetical commune described above, potent maternal bonding might make it more difficult for mothers to later lose interest in their child's well-being. A commune that really intended to hinder maternal interest might separate mothers and infants from the moment of birth to prevent the bonding process. But if for whatever reason commune birth practices allowed postpartum contact between mother and child, so that bonding could occur, then genes which strengthened bonding might decrease inclusive fitness. The reader will recall that, in the example given, mothers might harm their child by trying to be of assistance. Mothers bound to their children might have a hard time resisting desires to later offer them aid. Consequently, after many generations of commune life, genes that promote strong bonds might be replaced by genes that promote no bonding at all, perhaps through their effects on neuroendocrine systems. A disposition promoting adherence to one ESS, embodied in equation (2.1), would then have been supplanted by an innate disposition promoting adherence to another ESS, determined by commune theology.

Culture

To what extent are cultural forces capable of altering innate dispositions producing adherence to particular social patterns? Alternatively, to what extent do cultural forces "de-couple" dispositions from their consequent social patterns, so that the same dispositions no longer have the same effect as in the environment in which they evolved? If cultural forces generally alter innate dispositions, or if they radically change the social consequences of those dispositions, the conceptual value of ESS's would be thrown into doubt. Even if ancient ESS's have taken root in the gene pool, they would be of little consequence if the innate dispositions upon which they depend could be swept aside or nullified at a moment's notice. The hypothetical commune cited above seems to support that possibility since it showed that an ancient ESS can in theory be uprooted by a stable strategy originating in culture. Nor is it necessary to confine ourselves to hypothetical instances. It is easy to enumerate actual instances in which culture seems in conflict with innate dispositions affecting social behavior. This is the province of Freudian conflict theory and the basis for the Freudian view of neurosis.

Obviously, persons raised in different cultures behave in profoundly different ways. But in spite of its great diversity, human social behavior does seem to reveal certain ubiquitous patterns, and some of these, being ESSs, are innately probable strategies as defined in the previous section. Apparently, regardless of what may be theoretically possible, cultural forces neither sweep away most innate dispositions nor radically alter the social effects they have. Culture, in other words, must be rather conservative in the face of innate dispositions.

Actually, at least two forces protect innately probable strategies from radical cultural forces that otherwise might threaten them. First, the type of strategy discussed in following chapters has been so important to social life, and thus to inclusive fitness, that it tends to be overdetermined. Adherence to these strategies was probably so adaptive in the environment in which humans evolved that nature did not put all her eggs in one basket. Many innate dispositions contribute to adherence to each strategy, not just one or a few. So if culture overrides one disposition, or interferes with realization of another, or alters somewhat the social effect of a third, there are probably still more dispositions promoting adherence to the strategy in question. Cases where culture has chopped away so thoroughly at the roots of a strategy that an unusual number of persons fail to adhere to it, are especially interesting from a public health point of view, and from the point of view of psychiatric epidemiology. These are discussed in the following chapters. As the reader will see, a culture that uprooted a strategy altogether would produce a wholly insane population, at least in the technical sense of modern western psychiatry.

Second, according to theories of cultural evolution which account for cultural change by invoking "selective retention," culture itself is molded by the same type of dispositions that I have argued promote adherence to innately probable strategies. According to these theories, material, ecologic, and historical forces produce cultural variants, which are then selectively retained or discarded by individuals whose preferences are determined in part by their innate dispositions. Insofar as culture is shaped by innate dispositions, the extent of possible conflict between culture and disposition is necessarily decreased.

The first recognizable selective retention theories were outlined by Morgan (1890, 1892) and William James (1890) during the 19th Century. Baldwin (1897) raised issues concerning the true determinants of selective retention. These issues have resurfaced only very recently, in work by Boyd and Richerson (1985). In recent years, increasingly sophisticated variants of selective retention theories have been developed, and selective retention concepts have been applied to a wide range of cultural phenomena (see, for example, Alexander, 1979; Aoki, 1986; Barkow, 1989; Boyd and Richerson, 1985; Campbell, 1960; Durham, 1978; Feldman, et al., 1985; Kurland, 1979; Langton, 1979; Lopreato, 1984; Lumsden, 1985, 1988, 1989; MacDonald, 1989; Reynolds and Tanner, 1983; Richards, 1987; Richerson and Boyd, 1989). The best known modern version of selective retention theory was developed by Lumsden and Wilson (1981, 1983, 1985). Lumsden and Wilson described "epigenetic rules," akin to innate dispositions. Epigenetic, or developmental, rules are determined by innate perceptual processes, stimulus or aesthetic preferences, gestures, affects, and cognitive traits, among other characteristics (see Lumsden, 1988). According to Lumsden and Wilson, epigenetic rules affect the probability that given "culturgens"—which arise through processes intrinsic to culture itself—will be selectively kept in the cultural repertoire. Culturgens are basic cultural subunits, such as physical artifacts, social customs, acquired beliefs, ideas, myths, or religious practices. In effect, epigenetic rules exert an unending pressure on cultural choices, forcing them into channels congenial to dispositions that result from genes.

Of course, the situation is sufficiently complex that no short summary statement, appropriate to this book, can do justice to it. Cultural forms, or culturgens, selectively retained because of their apparent concordance with innate dispositions may have unforeseeable long-term effects at odds with these dispositions or with others. The automobile, for instance, caught on as a means of transportation because it satisfied numerous needs more or less related to innate dispositions. One of its long-term effects, though, was attenuation of family and neighborly ties. Due to their great mobility, many people today are out of touch with their families and don't even know their neighbors. As I will argue in later chapters, innate affective dispositions make people maintain contact with family and neighbors, so the automobile here has attenuated a social effect of an innate disposition. Other examples like this, and their effects on mental health, are discussed in later chapters.

Selective retention is also complicated by social inequities. Social and economic ideologies, sexual and moral injunctions, rules and taboos, and ideals of conduct and character are selectively retained or not along with more concrete cultural products (see Wolff, 1978; Markl, et al., 1978, for application of selective retention models to ethical ideology). But because ideologic, moral, and conduct control depend on potential punishment, only those able to impose or avoid punishment in any given society can selectively impose or discard cultural products of this sort. Therefore, selective retention of ideologies, mores, and ideals is a potent means by which the powerful in any given society can mold the behavior of the lower classes to promote their own interests, which manifest in part their innate dispositions (see Alexander, 1979; Breuer, 1982; Krebs, 1987; Kurland,

1979; N.W. Thornhill and Thornhill, 1987). Historians, of course, have always known that ethics can be and are used in this way. For example, Gibbon (quoted in Harrington, 1983) wrote of Roman religion:

> The various modes of worship which prevailed in the ancient world were all considered by the people as equally true; by the philosophers as equally false; and by the magistrates as equally useful.

This view is also central to Marxian ethical theory (see Sowell, 1985) and to feminist theory (see Dijkstra, 1986).

The peculiar position of ethics in selective retention theories, which makes it a tool for the powerful to advance their own interests, explains many instances where culture and innate dispositions seem to be in conflict. In these cases, the young, the weak, or the powerless are the ones whose dispositions are thwarted by cultural rules more favorable to those who impose and maintain them. For example, and of greatest interest from a strictly psychiatric viewpoint, specific parental injunctions serve to mold children's behavior in ways most advantageous to parental inclusive fitness. Children who rebel against these injunctions eventually impose them upon their own offspring. This is because their innate dispositions, reflecting altered inclusive fitness interests, change as they mature and eventually coincide with those that had once influenced their parents' moral preferences. Freud (1923) considered this process dependent on introjection of parental restraints. Sociobiological models do not predict the actual mechanism by which children adopt their parents mores. They only predict that the process will somehow occur.

Insofar as the powerful shape culture to control the weak, then much of the apparent conflict between culture and nature is actually a conflict between the weak and powerful, apotheosized in mores, punishments, and criminal acts visible to the outsider. And the interests of both the weak and powerful are shaped by innate dispositions interacting with differing exigencies. The situation gets even more complex when mores and ideals are shaped by more than one social class differing in their interests; ethical ideologies in this case might lack internal consistency.

Though selective retention theory helps to explain why ESS's survive in spite of cultural change, it should not be overrated as a theory of history. Societies have dynamics independent of choices made by particular actors (cf. Durkheim, 1950). To ignore these dynamics would lead us to overestimate biologic control over cultural change. Schmookler (1984), for instance, described one important dynamic independent of preferences based on innate dispositions. I will describe this here, since it will prove relevant to issues in later chapters.

According to Schmookler, the agricultural revolution, which was driven by population growth five or six thousand years ago, heightened intergroup conflict by raising the stakes involved. Formation of in-groups inimical to outsiders is an ancient ESS characteristic of humans (see chapter 5). But pre-agrarian peoples had little to gain from conflict. Consequently, conflicts between hunter-gatherer groups most likely were minor, as they are today. With agrarianism, this situation changed. Arable land and slaves could be obtained through warfare and justified its costs. According to Schmookler, prolonged and violent warfare selected among societies in the agrarian era. Due to an inexorable intergroup dynamic, only those societies efficiently geared for war have survived to the present day.

There are complications, too, to selective retention models that belie their apparent simplicity. Boyd and Richerson (1985) note that social modeling processes, and not just personal preferences, determine choices involved in selective retention. Boyd and Richerson show that cultural variants at odds with innate dispositions and disadvantageous to fitness may spread because of models that favor them in some way, or because of effects of conformity. Modeling and conformity are discussed in chapter 4.

As Boyd and Richerson predict, maladaptive cultural traits are in fact rather common. Reynolds and Tanner (1983), for instance, provide an exhaustive account of maladaptive behaviors, decreasing inclusive fitness, traceable just to religious beliefs. Some of these behaviors may result from types of selective retention described by Boyd and Richerson, but others may serve inclusive fitness interests of those in positions of power.

Issues of cultural history, and the biologic basis of culture, obviously cannot be resolved here. What is important for this study is that certain ESS's are in fact universal. This is in spite of whatever limitations exist to selective retention theories, and in spite of the possibilities for maladaptive behaviors due to societal factors. For reasons discussed above, universal ESS's are reasonably considered innately probable strategies. These strategies are described in the following chapters.

3
Parent-Child Relationships

Parental Altruism

Equation (2.1) describes a social strategy: provide aid to genetic kin whenever rB, the coefficient of relationship (r) times the benefit (B), exceeds C, the cost. Since r is always less than or equal to one, rB represents a depreciated benefit; the depreciation is greater the smaller the value of r, or the more distant the kinship. As discussed in the previous chapter, the "kin altruistic" strategy represented by equation (2.1) is evolutionarily stable. By definition, individuals adhering to alternative strategies would either provide aid when the cost exceeded the depreciated benefit or fail to provide aid when it would not. Unlike most evolutionarily stable strategies, the kin altruistic strategy retains its stability regardless of its frequency in the population.

Is the kin altruistic strategy also universal? Certainly, in all societies individuals are more willing to help other people when the cost-benefit ratio is low, as equation (2.1) requires. People are more likely to throw a rope than to jump into the water; they are more likely to aid someone who will benefit from their help than to aid someone who does not need assistance. Individuals everywhere also are eager to aid their closest genetic kin, as equation (2.1) requires.

The extent to which humans adhere to kin altruism in their relationships with distant relatives is clouded by the fact that some nominal kinship classifications, which ostensibly direct aid, fail to correspond to second and lesser degrees of genetic relatedness (see, for example, Sahlins, 1976). A number of authors have observed that nominal kinship systems serve not only altruistic, but economic, military, and sexual functions too (see, for example, Alexander,

1979; Chagnon, 1982; Chagnon and Irons, 1979; Fox, 1967, 1979, 1980; Levi-Strauss, 1969; N.W. Thornhill and Thornhill, 1987; van den Berghe, 1987). Some of the latter are best served by kinship classifications that are less than perfectly accurate in genetic terms. In fact, several cues may be used to detect genetic relatedness without recourse to kinship classifications (Blaustein, 1983; Holmes and Sherman, 1983; Porter, 1987; Rushton, et al., 1984; Smith 1988). These cues are apparently utilized by the many nonhuman primate and other animal species who engage in kin altruism, and some may be used by humans to direct altruistic behaviors regardless of kinship systems.

As a universal ESS, kin altruism meets the criteria described in the previous chapter for innately probable strategies.

Because the infant and young child need help to survive, efforts directed toward providing aid to an infant or young child are more beneficial to the recipient than equivalently costly efforts directed toward helping older children or adults. "B" in equation (2.1) which reflects the biologic value to the recipient of altruistic aid, is especially large for aid given to youngsters. Therefore, adults and older children should be ready to render aid to infants and small children to whom they are closely related. This is, of course, the case in all known societies. The most certain biologic relation is that between mother and child, so the mother in particular should be ready to help her infants and her young children. And in fact every culture respects the maternal caretaking role, at least in the early years of the child's life. This is all that is needed to set the stage for discussing relationships between parents and children.

Attachment

Mothers, and possibly other first or second degree biologic kin, adhere to the strategy embodied in equation (2.1) by maintaining attachment relationships with children. In psychiatry, Bowlby (1969, 1973, 1977, 1981) has argued persuasively for the importance of early attachment relationships to child behavior and mental and physical health. Adults, of course, are important in many diverse ways to infant and child mental well-being. For example, during much of the first year, frequent and somewhat stereotyped social interactions with adults are apparently needed for infant cognitive, affective, and social development. Very young infants deprived of sufficient attention may become unresponsive and literally waste away. But toward the end of the first year of life, the baby seems also to become "attached" to its accustomed caretakers who become its "attachment figures." The most important, or "principal" attachment figure for the child, is nearly always the mother. However, fathers or other family members may be the principal attachment figures in extraordinary circumstances, or may be "subsidiary attachment figures" ameliorating partially the effect of maternal absence. Fathers and other family members are more involved in child-rearing and consequently play more important attachment roles in certain tribal cultures than in Western societies (see, for example, Blain and Barkow, 1988). In what follows, I will generally refer to the principal attachment figure as the mother, in order to minimize jargon. The reader should keep in mind, though, that others may play this role.

Children seek aid from their attachment figures, who are generally eager to give it. In order to ensure the timely flow of aid, children and their attachment figures maintain close and continual proximity, as the term "attachment" implies. A mother, father, aunt, uncle, or sibling cannot leave a baby behind in the forest, for instance, and expect to be able to aid it in a timely fashion when it is hungry or cold or exposed to various dangers. Toddlers and older children take an active part in preventing separations. The distance maintained between children and their attachment figures is determined in part by the perceived likelihood that aid will be required. If separations develop when assistance might be needed, children and their attachment figures will actively seek the other. Children especially may show signs of very intense fearfulness, with behavioral inhibition, at unwanted separations (Bowlby, 1969).

Long-lasting disruptions of fully formed attachment relationships have adverse effects not seen following disruptions of less vital relationships. According to Bowlby (1969), the older infant or child enduring an unwanted and lengthy separation from his or her mother will protest more or less violently. The child might call or search for her, or try to enlist aid in helping to recover her. The child may be anxious just as it is during shorter separations (cf. Suomi, et al., 1981). After a few days, and especially if subsidiary attachment figures aren't available to ameliorate the child's distress, the child seems to despair. He or she becomes apathetic and withdrawn and gives up the various efforts to call to or find the mother. It is very hard for others to establish meaningful contact with the child, in spite of the fact that the child's acute distress seems to have lessened. The mother's return at this point, unlike during the stage when the child was still protesting, will probably not elicit clearcut signs of relief. The child is likely instead to be angry and rejecting. Obvious signs of affection and a desire for closeness will reemerge only gradually, when the anger has abated. Even lengthier absences will produce a state of "detachment." The child becomes docile but emotionally unreachable. Should the mother return, she is likely to be met with long-lasting indifference, interspersed with anger. The previous relationship may be slowly reestablished, or permanently altered in the severest cases.

Bowlby argues that long-lasting separations from the principal attachment figure in early childhood lead to developmental failures and to adult psychopathology. Mothers who lack affection, or who are mentally or physically ill may also harm their children even without separations. Bowlby argues, in effect, that the child's perceptions are as important as physical facts. The child who sees that his would-be attachment figure fails to act like an attachment figure should, and is inattentive or even indifferent to his needs and proximity, will be damaged much the same as the abandoned child.

Bowlby's emphasis on the psychological importance of the attachment relationship to the older infant and child, and on the consequences of its disruption, has stimulated research on responses to separation. The best known technique for studying such responses is the Ainsworth Strange Situation Test (see Ainsworth, 1982; Ainsworth, et al., 1978; Ainsworth and Wittig, 1969; Bretherton, 1985). The Strange Situation Test is applied to infants, usually between the ages of nine and eighteen months. Infants are given an opportunity to explore and play with toys in an unfamiliar playroom with their mother and an experimenter present. The same behaviors are observed with the mother absent. Ainsworth initially devised this test to observe the effect of maternal absence on exploratory behavior, but it soon became clear that the infant's behavior on the mother's return to the playroom was of even greater interest. Infants showed the same types of response to the mother as described by Bowlby after long separations. Some infants immediately returned to the mother or sought her attention. Others seemed angry with her and resistant to interaction; still others tried to ignore her. Infants could be classified according to their behavior following separations, and these classifications turned out to be highly stable. Recent research, using assessment techniques applicable to older children, has shown that early classifications on the Ainsworth Strange Situation Test performed with the mother accurately predict analogous classifications made many years later (see, for example, Main, et al., 1985). Ainsworth classifications in tests with the mother also predict coping skills and abilities at a much later date (Ainsworth, et al., 1978; Arend, et al., 1979; Bretherton, 1985; Egeland, 1983; Erickson, et al., 1985; Matas, et al., 1978; Sroufe, 1983; Sroufe, et al., 1984; Waters, et al., 1979). These skills and abilities are requisite to optimal psychosocial development; their relative deficit in children with "insecure" classifications on the Ainsworth Test, who resist or ignore the mother on her return, may produce psychological problems of the type discussed by Bowlby.

Studies have shown that mothers of insecure infants are less sensitive to their children's needs and emotional cues and are physically less expressive than mothers of other infants (Ainsworth, et al., 1978; Belsky, et al., 1984; Crockenberg, 1981; Grossmann, et al., 1985; Miyake, et al., 1985). Cultural factors influence both maternal behavior and the proportion of infants rated as insecure on the Ainsworth Test (Grossmann, et al., 1985, Miyake, et al., 1985; Sagi, et al., 1985). Attachment researchers speculate that postseparation responses reflect the infant's working model of the attachment figure, and of its relation to her, and serve a tactical function in light of that working model (see, for example, Main, et al., 1985). The working model is stable and accounts for long-term stability of reunion behavior. In positing working models, attachment researchers seem to be moving toward object-relational theories, which for a long time have been popular among clinicians (see, for example, Greenberg and Mitchell, 1983).

I have already noted that parental attachment behaviors subserve parental altruism. Parental altruism is innately probable (see above), so parental involvement in attachment relationships must be innately probable too. In prehistoric times, the inclusive fitness penalties incurred by parents, especially mothers, consequent on failure to establish attachment relationships must have been severe. Throughout human prehistory, youngsters deprived of timely aid no doubt quickly died or came to serious harm. Inclusive fitness penalties for failed attachment relationships would have led to selection for genes promoting closer attachment between parent and child.

Involvement in attachment relationships is also innately probable when viewed as a childhood strategy. First, it is universal. Normal children everywhere are parties to such relationships with caregiving figures. Second, it is an ESS. Children who manage to stay in an attachment relationship with a benevolent helper are clearly better off than children who lack an attachment relationship. Inclusive fitness disadvantages accruing to children who lack attachment relationships are also independent of the frequency of attachment relationships in the population.

There is an important difference between the view espoused here and the view presented by Bowlby (1969). I account for parent and child involvement in attachment relationships by citing inclusive fitness benefits accruing to parents and children. Bowlby (1969) invoked "group selection" to account for the same phenomena. He apparently was unaware of inclusive fitness at all. Hamilton (1964) had defined inclusive fitness only five years before Bowlby (1969) published the first part of what later became his trilogy. Bowlby argued, in effect, that the complementary activities of attachment figures and children serve to promote survival of the social group as a whole. Until very recently, many biologists accepted the view that natural selection of behavioral characteristics occurred at the level of groups (see Ghiselin, 1974; Lack, 1966; Maynard Smith, 1976b; Ruse, 1980; Wade, 1978; Williams, 1966; Wilson, 1980; Wynne-Edwards, 1962, 1963). This is called "group selection." According to this view, which is mostly discounted today, groups carrying genes conducive to adaptive behaviors have outcompeted other groups which eventually disappeared. Bowlby's use of group selection had important effects on his theory; these are described below.

Parents' Innate Dispositions
Promoting Attachment Relationships

Several known innate dispositions promote parental involvement in attachment relationships with young children. These are probably just the "tip of the iceberg"—at the present time, parental psychobiology is mostly terra incognita—but they are nonetheless worth mentioning here. Presumably, these dispositions evolved through selective advantages of adherence to the ESS expressed by equation (2.1).

I noted in chapter 2 that postpartum interaction with the newborn baby affects later maternal behavior. The postpartum period appears to be "critical," in the sense that long-term maternal caretaking behaviors are affected by interactions during a rather short time span. Interrupting postpartum contact between mother and infant seems to decrease later maternal warmth and sensitivity to the child (see Ali and Lowry, 1981; Carlsson, et al., 1978; DeChateau and Wiberg, 1977a, 1977b; Hales, et al., 1977; Klaus, et al., 1972; O'Connor, et al., 1977; Trowell, 1982). Maternal warmth and sensitivity predict attachment behaviors observed in the Ainsworth Test (Ainsworth, et al., 1978; Belsky, et al., 1984; Crockenberg, 1981; Grossmann, et al., 1985; Miyake, et al., 1985). These in turn predict childhood coping skills (Ainsworth, et al., 1978; Arend, et al., 1979; Bretherton, 1985; Egeland, 1983; Erickson, et al., 1985; Matas, et al., 1978; Sroufe, 1983; Sroufe, et al., 1984; Waters, et al., 1979). Thus, the events of a few days have widening repercussions. Diminished postpartum contact may even produce maternal neglect (see O'Connor, et al., 1977; Trowell, 1982). As noted in chapter 2, the mother's postpartum receptiveness to her infant may depend on physiologic processes associated with delivery, such as hormonal changes.

During the postpartum critical period, the mother learns to identify her infant, both by sight and sound. This is of obvious value for later provision of aid. Hours after giving birth, mothers can identify photographs of their newborn infant's face (Porter, et al., 1984), or their newborn infant's odor (Porter, et al., 1983; Russell, et al., 1983). Morsbach and Bunting (1979) found that twenty-two of twenty-seven mothers three to eight days postpartum could identify their newborns by the sound of their voices alone. Discriminant skills of this type, acquired without conscious effort, depend on innate nervous processes. Odor cues may be determined by histocompatibility genes (Yamaguchi, et al., 1981).

Perceptual dispositions produce caretaking behaviors. For example, adults enjoy viewing "cute" infants and children. That infants and children are fun to watch is obviously significant with regard to proximity maintenance. Increased relative head size and foreshortened facial features are important discriminant cues affecting perceived "cuteness." Lorenz (1981) argued that increased head size and foreshortened facial features comprise an innate "releaser" for human parental responses (see also Gardner and Wallach, 1965). Dolls and stuffed animals with enlarged heads and small facial features, or pictures depicting them, are sold for decorations. They are said to be cute, and they provide enough pleasure that people pay to have them. Females in particular admit to enjoying cuteness. Males may enjoy it as much but deny it to save face. Babyish smiles and vocalizations, and awkward, uncertain movements (Lorenz, 1981), produce the same responses as foreshortened faces and head size.

Affects also promote adult attachment behaviors. Parents love their child. Uncertainty about their child's safety makes them anxious. Injury to their child makes them feel distressed. The distress is ameliorated by seeing the child recover. Limbic brain structures apparently generate emotional experiences, or at least these structures ensure they occur at appropriate times (Berger and Brodie, 1986). Brain structure, in turn, reflects genetic activity.

Infant distress vocalizations elicit adult autonomic responses and subjective arousal (Donovan, et al., 1978). Physiologic responses may be preparatory: they may ready the adult to provide aid to the infant. In any event, they are likely to intensify or alter parental moods (cf. Erdman and Janke, 1978; Schachter and Singer, 1962; Schacter and Wheeler, 1962; Valins, 1966), so as to alter behavior in an adaptive fashion. Physiologic response patterns to infant vocalizations are probably also innate, or depend on innate mechanisms.

Finally, parental motoric and communicative dispositions work to favor attachment. Some of these dispositions seem to be innate. For example, in chapter 2 I noted the infant's attentiveness to the human face and voice. Infantile responsiveness predicts later behavior in the Strange Situation Test (Grossmann, et al., 1985). Without making conscious efforts, parents behave in such a way as to increase infant responsiveness. For instance, they hold infants so as to show their faces in the proper orientation and at the proper distance to catch the infant's attention (Stern, 1977, 1985). They exaggerate gestures, alter their voices, and change their pattern of speech (Papousek and Papousek, 1979; Snow, 1972; Stern, 1977, 1985; Stern, et al., 1982; Trevarthen, 1979).

Adults also unconsciously provide motoric, vocal, and facial expressive feedback that alters the infants' affective state and consequent proximity maintenance (see below).

Studies of carrying styles show how parental dispositions can mold the attachment relationship. Salk (1973) found that both right- and left-handed mothers most often carry their newborn infant in such a way that the infant's head lies on their left breast. When carried in this position, the newborn hears the mother's heart, which has a calming effect. In the environment in which human behavior evolved, mothers with calmer neonates may have had an incremental survival advantage. Or it may have been advantageous to the newborn to be calm. In any event, the mother's ability to soothe her infant is an important element of the attachment relationship, and partly determines—through its effect on the mother's as well as the infant's affect—the course it will take. So a simple motor disposition—affecting how the infant is carried—might incrementally alter the fate of a long-term relationship. Evidence points toward an innate component to this disposition: the preference discovered by Salk is manifested cross-culturally (Lockhard, et al., 1979); it is shown in works of art from many historical periods (Finger, 1975). Significantly, it may fail to develop if mother and neonate are separated during the immediate postpartum period (Trowell, 1982). Maternal anxiety may have the same effect (DeChateau, 1983). Males and females differ in the way they carry things. Women more often carry objects against their breast, the way they carry infants; men more often carry objects with their hands, their arms hanging at their sides. These differences develop before adolescence, so they cannot be attributed solely to anatomic differences between the sexes (Jenni and Jenni, 1976).

Children's Innate Dispositions Promoting
Attachment Relationships

In this section, too, I provide a few examples, which are only the tip of the iceberg. These help to show how innate dispositions promote adherence to strategies.

Infants and children rely on their parents. In order for them to survive, the parents or other adults must keep them close at hand and provide them with aid. But dependency in this case isn't the same as passivity. Infants and children aren't passive. Even the newborn, helpless in other respects, exerts some degree of control over caretaking parents. The control exercised by infants and children is not always, or even usually, volitional. Without volitional effort, infant and child dispositions may interact with the parent's to promote parental aid and attachment behaviors. For example, I have already mentioned the infant's attentiveness to faces (see chapter 2). This is apparent shortly after birth and therefore must be innate. The infant's attention to faces promotes face-to-face contact with parents or other adults. With face-to-face contact, the infant's immature features elicit positive feelings from observing adults: the attentive infant is "cute" (see above). These feelings reinforce adult goodwill and proximity maintenance. Similar remarks apply to the newborn's attentiveness to the sound of the human voice, and to the sound of the mother's voice (see chapter 2), which he or she heard in the womb. The newborn's attentiveness to adult faces and voices help it to "seduce" adults into attachment relationships.

Innate gestures and vocalization also help the infant and child. I noted in chapter 2 that universally understood facial gestures appear shortly after birth. They develop in blind infants, so they cannot be imitations. They appear to function as positive or negative reinforcers for parents who respond to them in a stereotyped, mostly unconscious fashion (Papousek and Papousek, 1979; Trevarthen, 1979). I noted above that the sound of a youngster crying can produce physiological arousal. Other immature vocalizations produce more pleasant feelings. Simply by making faces or noise the infant or child can therefore reinforce greater degrees of parental aid and proximity-maintenance.

As children mature, they not only manage their caretakers, they

take a more direct approach to parental aid and proximity maintenance. First, they cling to the mother and—in many "primitive"
societies—spend long hours at the breast, sucking intermittently.
Similar behaviors are shown by nonhuman primates. Bowlby (1969)
has argued that the child's desire to cling and suck are innate; long
periods at the mother's breast being the highly adaptive norm except
in modern societies. According to Bowlby, these desires account for
so-called transitional objects. In societies that limit the child's opportunities for clinging and sucking, inanimate objects with sufficient
morphologic and textural similarities to the mother's body may
become targets of clinging and sucking behaviors which would
otherwise have been directed her way. Well used transitional objects
also have an odor that enhances their desirability to the child. Odor
appears more important in determining social behavior of human
infants than has previously been acknowledged (see, for example,
MacFarlane, 1975; Russell, 1976). Consistent with Bowlby's suggestion, transitional objects are more likely to be used by small
children if the mother is absent or unavailable, or if the child is tired,
ill, or frightened. Harlow's well-known studies (e.g. Harlow, 1971;
Harlow and Zimmerman, 1959; Harlow, et al., 1971) showed that
the harmful effects of maternal deprivation could be mitigated for
nonhuman primates, specifically rhesus monkeys, by providing what
were apparently transitional objects. These satisfied the infant's
desire to cling or suck despite the mother's absence. Though the issue
is outside my purview here, the reader should note that Bowlby's
account of transitional objects is not necessarily inconsistent with
Winnicott's (1958) germinal viewpoint (see also Davis and Wallbridge, 1981). Instead, Bowlby and Winnicott address different
aspects, ethologic and intrapsychic, of the same phenomenon.

Once they are able to ambulate, young children assume more
and more of the burden for active proximity maintenance. Social
and cultural factors affect the degree of responsibility for proximity
maintenance borne by children of any age, but in most societies,
children of four or five assume a significant share of it. Childhood
dispositions promote active efforts to remain near the parents. Two
especially important ones, at least from a clinical viewpoint, are the
child's desire to obtain parental attention and the child's affective
responses to separation and strangers.

Toddlers and young children seek parental attention. The manner in which they do so varies from culture to culture, even from family to family. In general though, from the time they are able to ambulate, children intermittently seek the parent to display their current activities and their most recent accomplishments. Kohut (1971, 1977) and his followers (see Goldberg, 1978, 1980) relate childhood self-display to narcissistic features of the adult personality (see chapter 4). In particular, parental failure to respond to the child's seemingly narcissistic needs for self-display are thought by Kohut and others to produce nacissistic pathology. Suffice it to say here that, quite aside from their relation to later self-regard, the narcissistic wishes displayed by the child also serve proximity maintenance. To satisfy these wishes, which Kohut thinks are universal, the parent must come to the child or the child must go to the parent. The net effect of these wishes then, from the standpoint of proximity maintenance, is to narrow the distance between parent and child.

Small children also depend on parental responses to judge unfamiliar stimuli or unfamiliar events (Campos and Stenberg, 1980; Emde and Sorce, 1983; Emde, et al., 1978). By calling parental attention to his or her current activities, the small child helps ensure that the parent will protect it from potential unknown dangers. In middle class society, it is easy to underestimate the potential dangers encountered by the youngster who lacked any desire to "show off" what he was doing. Middle class children are raised today in "child-proofed" houses; these reduce the adaptive value of calling parental attention to every new activity.

I have already noted the "separation anxiety" children apparently feel when deprived of ready access to their mother or other attachment figure (see Bowlby, 1969). As expected, given that the adaptive function of proximity maintenance resides in greater access to parental aid, factors that imply an increased need for parental aid increase the intensity of separation anxiety. Hunger, fatigue, or illness, for instance, increase the anxiety produced by decreased access to an attachment figure. Separation anxiety reinforces the child's efforts to maintain proximity to his attachment figures.

In humans, segments of the Ainsworth Strange Situation Test during which the mother is absent have been used to measure separation anxiety. Anxious children, for instance, decrease play and exploration during the mother's absence (Ainsworth and Wittig, 1969; Cox and Campbell, 1968). In general, it may be possible to conceptualize anxiety as a subjective correlate of behavioral inhibition, the latter being adaptive in certain situations (see Fischman, et al., 1977; Howard and Pollard, 1977). In animals, separation anxiety has been studied pharmacologically (see, for example, Fabre-Nys, et al., 1982; Kraemer and McKinney, 1979; McKinney, 1985, 1988; Panksepp, et al., 1978) and physiologically (see, for example, Coe and Levine, 1981; Levine, 1982; McKinney, 1985, 1988; Reite, et al., 1981).

Even if they have not had any traumatic experience with unfamiliar persons, small children are often frightened by adult strangers, especially males (Bronson, 1972; Smith, 1979; Waters, et al., 1975). Psychological theories of childhood stranger anxiety have generally failed to take account of its real adaptive value. Unfamiliar adults, males in particular, pose a threat to infants in modern-day primate species (see, for example, Hrdy, 1974, 1977, 1981; Kummer, et al., 1974; Sugiyama, 1967). They likely posed a similar threat in protohominid species. When frightened by a stranger, the typical child quickly moves in its mother's direction. The antidote to stranger anxiety seems to be contact with mother. In fact, once in contact with mother, many children will seem not to be frightened at all by those they have just run away from. Once again anxiety reinforces proximity maintenance and consequently attachment.

Situation-specific aid seeking and anxiety indicate, of course, that the infant considers himself somehow inadequate to deal with certain exigencies without adult assistance (see below).

Positive feeling states attendant on proximity to the attachment figure are much less well characterized, both descriptively and in terms of their correlates, than negative feeling states attendant on separation. Negative feelings have proven easier to study. Positive feeling states which may promote proximity-maintenance include feelings of love for the mother, feelings of safety and security, and perhaps so-called "oceanic feelings" (see Fenichel, 1945).

Like parental love, filial love must be largely innate. If nothing else, innate mechanisms that direct the child's attention to its fellow human beings and permit communication with them increase the odds that the child will form affective ties to the parents, since the parents are more or less constantly present. If Freud (1940) was correct, innate bodily drives also play an important role, at least in love of the mother. The mother feeds the infant and meets his bodily needs. Because she is repeatedly associated with bodily satisfaction, the mother, according to Freud, eventually comes to be wished for regardless of bodily state (cf. Hartmann (1952, 1953) on "object constancy"). In learning theory terms, the mother becomes a secondary reward, bodily needs being primary. Since Freud, however, even psychoanalysts have been split on the role of bodily drives in very early feelings of love (Greenberg and Mitchell, 1983). Fairbairn's ideas on the primacy of loving relationships paved the way for attachment theory in its present form (Fairbairn, 1952; Guntrip, 1961, 1971). Various empirical studies have also weakened Freud's argument for the importance of bodily drives. Both primate and human infants can develop apparently typical filial feelings for maternal surrogates who never address their bodily needs (Ainsworth, 1963; Bowlby, 1958, 1969; Harlow, 1971; Harlow and Zimmerman, 1959; Harlow, et al., 1971; Schaffer and Emerson, 1964; Stevens, 1982). In fact, feelings might run deeper when bodily needs are involved; the evidence indicates only that bodily needs aren't required for some form of love to emerge. Freud's theory is incomplete, but it may not be completely wrong.

In the foregoing sections, I have argued that various dispositions enhance the probability that parent and child will become parties to an attachment relationship. I have cited some dispositions that plausibly seem to be wholly or partly innate. I have not found need to mention any organizational process above and beyond dispositions. Bowlby (1969), on the other hand, argues that the child's aid seeking and proximity maintenance is under feedback control of an attachment "system." He sees in the child's behavior an overall organization, such that corrective processes are activated when aid is inadequate or proximity maintenance fails. Where Bowlby views attachment as the result of feedback to an organized system, I have portrayed it here as the more or less incidental result of varying dispositions, which have as their "side effects" the ready flow of aid and increased physical closeness.

The child acts, of course, in an apparently purposeful way. But the child's apparent purposefulness does not require that we postu-

late an overall organizational scheme above and beyond dispositions. "Blind" dispositions, especially contingent ones, can produce
apparently goal-directed behaviors without superordinate feedback
loops or executive systems. That is why dispositions evolved. Many
social relationships—including adult ones—are formed "inciden-
tally," due to dispositions.

Parent-Child Conflict and Discriminative Parenting

The child differs genetically from either of its parents. Consequently, the child's inclusive fitness interests are capable of conflict-
ing with the interests of either parent. There are two basic types of
parent-child conflict, and both of these are important in theories of
psychopathology. Bowlby (1969) recognized that parent-child conflict occurs, but he could not account for it because he had adopted
a group-selectionist framework. That is, he saw attachment relationships as good for the group or species, not as a strategy created
by individual needs. At the time Bowlby developed his ideas, group-
selectionist theories were the major means of accounting for altruistic behaviors (see above). "Inclusive fitness" was coined in 1964
(Hamilton, 1964), only five years before *Attachment* (Bowlby,
1969) was published. Detailed inclusive fitness accounts of parent-
child relationships first appeared after Bowlby (1969, 1973) had
published the first two volumes of *Attachment and Loss.* Insofar as
parents and children develop attachment relationships for the good
of group or species—and not to increase inclusive fitness—then it is
hard to see why conflicts might arise between them. Insofar as they
cooperate for the good of the group, for example, parent and child
must have identical interests.

The first and most important type of parent-child conflict occurs
when the child seeks more aid than the parent wants to provide. The
coefficient of relationship between parent and child is only 0.5.
Simple rearrangements of equation (2.1) show that parents and children who maximize inclusive fitness will disagree whether aid
should be given whenever the ratio of parental cost to child benefit
is moderately high. If prospective parental costs become even higher
relative to benefits, parent and child interests once again converge.
Readers interested in the details of this argument are referred to
Trivers (1974). A well-known objection raised to Trivers's argu-

ment (Alexander, 1974) has been shown to be incorrect (Blick, 1977; MacNair and Parker, 1978; Metcalf, et al., 1979; O'Connor, 1978; Parker and MacNair, 1978; Stamps, et al., 1978).

As noted in chapter 2, inclusive fitness theories imply no calculations; in this case neither child nor parent has heard of inclusive fitness. Instead, insofar as predictable stratagems maximized inclusive fitness for ancestral humans, innate dispositions promoting their realization must have been selected for. These dispositions are with us today, affecting social behavior. For example, today's child might be predisposed to ask for slightly more aid than the parent seems willing to give; today's parent might be predisposed to give slightly less aid than the child seems to want.

The infant, of course, is in no position to press his case too far. But as the child grows, he becomes increasingly able to express dissatisfaction with parental care. Bowlby (1973) and others (see, for example, Ainsworth, 1982; Ainsworth, et al., 1978 on type C attachments; George and Main, 1979) describe childhood anger in response to what the child perceives as inadequate care. Every parent knows how stridently children may press for more aid and assistance than parents prefer to give. Conflicts over parental aid have been described as well in nonhuman primate species (see, for example, Hinde and Spencer-Booth, 1967, 1971; Rosenblum, 1971; Struhsaker, 1971).

Insofar as parental aid adheres to equation (2.1), it is under control of factors affecting cost-benefit ratios. By controlling parental aid, these factors also regulate parent-child conflicts. For example, parents with abundant physical and social resources can provide aid to their children at less cost to themselves than parents without resources. Very high rates of parental aid due to parental resources should alleviate conflicts between parent and child. Conversely, low rates due to lack of resources should exacerbate conflicts. Very severe conflicts between parents and children associated with poverty have in fact been described (see, for example, Hippler, 1974). Differences in the intensity of parent-child conflicts could affect personality structure and contribute to social class differences in rates of psychopathology (see below). Parents are also sensitive to fluctuations in need for aid, and consequently in benefits. They are more willing to provide aid at times when aid might be crucial. In order to obtain more aid, children alert their parents to dangers, illness, or injuries that increase their need for assistance. Unhappy with what they perceive as waning parental attention, children may mimic neediness. Feigned illness or injury, false incapacity or immaturity, or exaggerated fearfulness all may be used by a child to bolster parental interest (see Trivers, 1974).

Parent-child conflicts may become more intense as the child develops new competencies. These may lead the parent to believe that the child needs less aid, while the child remains uncertain of his new capacities. The "separation-individuation" process, which Mahler, Pine, and Bergman (1975) argue is important to later development, is obviously comprised in part of parent-child conflicts intensified by the child's growing motor competence in its second year.

Child-rearing practices affecting intensity of parent-child conflicts probably partly determine culture-specific differences in personality types (Erikson, 1950; Konner, 1982) and religious beliefs (Lambert, et al., 1959; Spiro and D'Andrade, 1958).

The second type of parent-child conflict concerns sibling relationships. Equation (2.1) predicts that children maximizing their own inclusive fitness will be modestly altruistic to nonidentical siblings. But simple transformations of equation (2.1) show that parental genes benefit from higher levels of intersibling altruism than those advantageous to the child. Readers interested in the details of this argument are referred once again to Trivers (1974). The argument depends on the fact that parents are equally related to each of their children; they should therefore maximize the average, rather than just individual, reproductive success attained by their children. Each child, on the other hand, should maximize his own inclusive fitness, and not the average reproductive success attained by his sibling group. Parent-child conflicts over sibling relationships may or may not be psychologically important. Once again, cultural and economic circumstances are likely determining factors. These affect the number of siblings and the costs and benefits accruing from sibling aid. If conflict is salient, it is likely waged by parents on an ideologic plane, with ethical injunctions promoting "brotherly love" (cf. chapter 2). That is because the parent desires not only to change the child's immediate behavior—for which coercion alone would suffice— but to change the child's behavior after it has grown, when the parent may be dead.

Clinicians often encounter individuals who report that their parents devalued them in comparison with their siblings. In many cases, these reports are probably exaggerated. I have noted above that even unbiased parents may not provide the aid a child wants to receive, and at the same time they may pressure the child to be more altruistic toward its siblings. Even-handed parental behaviors might be selectively distorted by individuals who feel deprived, to establish their claim that their siblings received favored treatment. On the other hand, inclusive fitness models do predict that parents may treat their children in greatly disparate fashion if parental investments in different children may produce greatly disparate effects on inclusive fitness. The most extreme example of "discriminative parenting," as it has been called, is selective infanticide. The selectively infanticidal parent chooses to cut off parental investments for some children altogether, in order to have more available to others. In several societies, selective infanticide shows a class distribution consistent with predictions made by inclusive fitness models (Dickemann, 1979; Voland, 1984). Though they condemn infanticide, most societies allow or encourage parents to discriminate to some degree among their various children (Daly and Wilson, 1980, 1981, 1982; Smith, 1988; Wilson, et al., 1981). Female children, especially, tend to be devalued in societies dominated by powerful males. Paternal aid in particular may be contingent on perceived similarity, which is a clue to paternity. Fathers who make large parental investments may discriminate in favor of children they perceive to be like them, at the expense of children they perceive as different. In chapter 5, I note that identification may be the psychological mechanism responsible for altruistic behavior in human beings. Every clinician has met fathers who identify with some of their children because of perceived similarities.

The Natural History of Attachment
and Models of Self and Others

Social strategies aimed at obtaining aid from and maintaining proximity to a caretaking figure are salient in childhood but become less evident with maturity. For example, as children become less depen-dent on a caretaker's constant assistance, exigencies eliciting obvi-ous aid and proximity seeking become more unusual. By the time they are full grown, normal persons manifest childlike attachment behavior in response to traumatic events, but not in more usual cir-cumstances. Bowlby (1973) noted that childlike attachment behav-iors are shown by adults following public disasters.

Many of the perceptual, cognitive, and affective processes that promote formation of childhood attachment relationships subserve different strategies in adult life. Others, such as intense fearfulness in unfamiliar settings, are normally attenuated. In the following sections, I will try to demonstrate that certain mental disorders result from abnormal salience during adult life of psychological processes subserving early attachment, or from abnormal salience of childlike attachment strategies considered as a whole. Psychological processes and attachment strategies may remain excessively salient because of genetic or biological factors or because of early expe-riences in attachment relationships. For example, studies of non-human primates (Hinde and Spencer-Booth, 1971; Spencer-Booth and Hinde, 1971a) and of humans (Brown, 1982; Brown, et al., 1977) suggest that disruptions of infant care-seeking strategies—by maternal deprivation, for instance—increase sensitivity to later stressful events, which are then more likely to elicit care-seeking behaviors.

Early attachment experiences might affect adult behaviors in at least two ways. First, early attachment relationships seem to pro-duce long-lasting expectations concerning how others behave, espe-cially those others on whom one might depend for assistance or affection (see, for example, Main, et al., 1985). For example, Miller (1981) described how children raised by narcissistic parents—who attend to their children only if they are "special"—come to believe that other persons will care for them only insofar as they are exceed-ingly bright, talented, or successful. They grow up to be driven and in need of reassurance that others perceive their talents. Likewise, many uninterested parents direct attention to children only if children forcefully breach their indifference. Children raised by these parents oftentimes grow up to be histrionic or angry. For them, anger and histrionics are means for securing attention. Children abandoned by parents often grow up believing that others will leave them too.

Second, interactions with parents and other attachment figures may alter later behavior through their effects on self-confidence. Both ethologists and psychologists have focused attention on the critical role of self-confidence in shaping behavior patterns. Parker (1974), for example, used the term "resource holding power" or (RHP) to refer to an individual's ability to compete with others for contested resources. He showed that subjective estimates of RHP determine responses to conflict. Individuals who can accurately estimate their RHP are better adapted, in an inclusive fitness sense, than individuals who cannot estimate RHP. In human groups, conflicts are most often fought in the social arena, not in physical combat. Consequently, human RHP is less dependent on physical size and strength than on social skills and position. In a previous work, I argued that determinants of human RHP are also the major determinants of self-esteem (Wenegrat, 1984). For example, attractiveness, prestige, wealth, charisma, and various skills increase self-esteem as well as RHP. Both self-esteem and RHP increase with successes in the social realm, and failures lower RHP and self-esteem together. I suggested that self-esteem is the subjective counterpart to RHP. More recently, Glantz and Pearce (1989) argued that self-esteem is the subjective counterpart to "dominance," a term I prefer to avoid in reference to human groups because of its connotations.

In recent years, many psychotherapists and cognitive psychologists have emphasized the importance of how people see their own competencies (see, for example, Abramson, et al., 1978; Bandura, 1977; Bandura, et al., 1977; Beck, 1972, 1976; Beck, et al., 1974; Costello, 1978; Ellis, 1962; Ellis and Grieger, 1977; Rizley, 1978; Seligman, 1975; Weintraub, et al., 1974). Bandura (1977), for instance, has argued that what he has called "self-efficacy"—a subjective belief in one's competence to master a situation—is needed for adaptations of widely varying kinds. Since the situations humans need to master are almost always social and involve potential conflicts over control of resources, self-efficacy in practice must be closely related to subjective RHP, and thereby to self-esteem.

Many psychoanalysts have noted the connection of self-esteem, and in effect, self-efficacy, to early relations with parents (see, for example, Brenner, 1974; Fenichel, 1945; Goldberg, 1978, 1980; Greenberg and Mitchell, 1983; Kohut, 1971, 1977; Mitchell, 1988). Human parental behaviors—especially provision of contingent reinforcement and responses to conflicts—seem well suited to lay the groundwork for the developing child's subjective RHP, self-esteem, or self-efficacy. Parent-child conflicts are discussed in the previous section. Contingent reinforcement—or reinforcement that varies with the infant's own behavior—has been shown to be needed by nonhuman primate infants to develop normal exploratory and problem-solving behaviors (Lewis and Goldberg, 1969; Mason, 1979; Watson, 1971). Animals raised without contingent reinforcement seem to lack confidence that they can affect their environment. Artificial provision of contingent reinforcement can ameliorate in part adaptive deficits shown by primates raised alone (for descriptions of these deficits, see Hinde and Spencer-Booth, 1971; Spencer-Booth and Hinde, 1971a). Although most human adults unconsciously respond to infant vocalizations, facial expressions, and movements in such a way as to provide maximal reinforcement (Brazelton, et al., 1975; Papousek and Papousek, 1979; Snow, 1972; Stern, 1977, 1985; Stern et al., 1982; Trevarthen, 1979), occasional parents tend to be unresponsive (see, for example, Ainsworth, et al., 1978; Belsky, et al., 1984; Crockenberg, 1981; Grossman, et al., 1985; Miyake, et al., 1985). Depressed parents, especially, are likely to be less responsive to infant and child behaviors. Parental unresponsiveness may account for the high incidence of psychological problems in children of depressives (Beardslee, et al., 1983; Parker, 1983; Pound, 1982; Sameroff, et al., 1982), quite independently of genetic factors.

Whatever its cause, low subjective RHP, self-esteem, or self-efficacy might lead to later problems in conflict situations, as Parker's models indicate. This is discussed further in the next chapter. It might also produce more salient attachment-related behaviors in adult life. Situationally specific lack of self-confidence is a potent trigger for attachment-related behaviors in young children, as well as a manifestation of adherence to attachment strategies (see above). Bowlby's (1973) observations on childlike attachment behaviors in adults who have survived catastrophes suggest that loss of self-confidence can activate attachment–seeking behaviors in adults as well. If nothing else, individuals with low estimates of their RHP, or with poor self-esteem or self-efficacy, are more likely to experience their current problems as personally unmanageable, and therefore to manifest attachment–related behaviors. Contrariwise, the development of normal adult self-esteem, self-efficacy, or subjective RHP might be a critical factor in—and not just a sign of—the decreased salience of childlike attachment strategies as individuals mature.

Agoraphobia

The agoraphobic patient cannot leave a familiar location, such as his home, and venture into public areas without risk of suffering from anxiety. In the home he is generally symptom-free. In public areas, he can be safe from anxiety only if closely accompanied by a familiar person he has come to trust (see Hallam, 1985; Marks, 1987; Mathews, et al., 1981). The agoraphobic, in effect, is behaving much like a child, who suffers from anxiety in unfamiliar places and around strangers in the absence of an attachment figure. Readers should recall the Ainsworth Strange Situation Test (see above). Children taking the Ainsworth Strange Situation Test are separated from their mother in an unfamiliar room with a stranger present. They manifest anxiety in several observable ways. In a familiar setting, such as the home, and without strangers present, children are generally untroubled by brief maternal absences.

The familiar persons on whom agoraphobics come to depend to leave their homes are nearly always benign and helpful figures suited to play an attachment role. In some cases they find themselves acting as full time attendants. If they withdraw or become angry, the agoraphobic patient is likely to feel more anxious.

Many, but not all, agoraphobics experience their anxiety in the form of panic attacks, which are severe anxiety states Bowlby (1973) and others (see, for example, Klein, 1980) believe resemble the separation anxiety states shown by young children. Although many studies do suggest that panic attacks differ pharmacologically and physiologically from milder states of anxiety and resemble separation anxiety states (see, for example, Fyer and Sandberg, 1988; Gittelman and Klein, 1973, 1984; Gorman, et al., 1984; Griez and Van den Hout, 1983; Grosz and Farmer, 1972; Grunhaus, et al.,

1981; Kelly, et al., 1971; Liebowitz, et al., 1984; Pitts and McClure, 1967; Rifkin, et al., 1981; Shear and Fyer, 1988; Sheehan, et al., 1980; Tyrer and Steinberg, 1975; Tyrer, et al., 1973; Zitrin, et al., 1980; Zitrin, et al., 1983), neither pharmacologic nor physiologic findings are essential to the point I am making here. For the present purposes, the important parallel between childhood separation and stranger anxieties on the one hand and agoraphobic anxiety on the other is that they are triggered by similar situations. This suggests that agoraphobia may be due to a resurgence, in adult life, of an affective process normally reinforcing early attachment relationships.

Some agoraphobics may display more generalized attachment-related behaviors, and not just anxiety symptoms. Panic disorder patients, many of whom go on to develop the full blown agoraphobic syndrome, are frequently rather dependent, aid-seeking personalities, even when their anxiety has been successfully treated (Green and Curtis, 1988; Reich and Troughton, 1988). Many panic patients suffer severe depressions (Grunhaus, 1988; Lesser, et al., 1988; Norton, et al., 1986). In the following section, I argue that persons prone to develop depressive illness characteristically seek childlike attachment relationships.

Genetic family studies are consistent with the hypothesis that factors promoting the agoraphobic syndrome affect processes related to attachment. Anxiety syndromes, agoraphobia, depression, borderline personality, and other illnesses referable to the exigencies of attachment (see below) tend to be found together in afflicted families (see, for example, Andrulonis, et al., 1981; Carey, 1982; Coryell, 1981; Insel and Murphy, 1981; Leckman, et al., 1983; Loranger, et al., 1982; Marks, 1969, 1987; Murray and Reveley, 1981; Rasmussen and Tsuang, 1986; Soloff and Millward, 1983; Stone, 1980). As a group, children of agoraphobics have been found to be more inhibited in unfamiliar settings than children of normal controls (Rosenbaum, et al., 1988). Behavioral inhibition in unfamiliar settings is thought to manifest separation anxiety. Along the same lines, children of agoraphobics more often have school phobias than children of normal controls (Berg, 1976; Weissman, et al., 1984). According to Bowlby (1973), school phobias manifest problems with attachment relationships.

In the previous section, I noted that problems in early relationships might lead to later problems with attachment. In fact, many agoraphobics report having had school phobias or severe childhood fears related to separations (Berg, et al., 1974; Deltito, et al., 1986; Klein, 1964; Zitrin and Ross, 1988). According to Bowlby (1973) and others (see, for example, Faravelli, et al., 1985; Roberts, 1964; Roth, 1959, 1960; Schapira, et al., 1970; Snaith, 1968), many agoraphobics have suffered early losses or other traumatic disturbances of attachment relationships. Other studies, though, fail to confirm any unusual patterns in early life histories of agoraphobic patients (see, for example, Arrindell, et al., 1983; Buglass, et al., 1977; Parker, 1979a; Thyer, et al., 1985). Similarly mixed findings have been reported by studies relating other disorders to early life experiences (see below). Part of the problem may be that somewhat elusive aspects of early attachment relationships, such as the quality of interactions with attachment figures, may be more important than more readily measured events, such as divorces or deaths, and may even mediate their effects on later disorders (see, for example, Breier, et al., 1988; Parker, 1979b, 1981, 1983).

Panic disorders and the agoraphobic syndrome frequently develop shortly following losses or other stressful events (Barlow, 1988; Faravelli and Pallanti, 1989; Last, et al., 1984; Roy-Byrne, et al., 1986). Some of these events may represent disruptions of existing relationships that have a prominent attachment-like element. Others may exacerbate a sense of vulnerability, and thereby incite more attachment behaviors. In light of the interrelation of childlike attachment and decreased self-efficacy, self-esteem, and subjective RHP (see above), it is particularly striking that recent therapeutic approaches to agoraphobia and to panic disorders stress decreased self-efficacy as an important factor (Barlow, 1988; Williams, 1987, 1988).

Chronic Mourning and Depression

Bowlby (1980) noted that adult mourning—which can occur following many types of losses—resembles behavior of children separated from parents. In particular, the initial angry denial and subsequent depression in the course of adult mourning resemble the stages of protest, despair, and detachment described in an earlier section. Physiologic changes observed in human depression, which Gray (1978) claimed might serve an adaptive function by producing hypoactivity, resemble similar changes shown by nonhuman primate infants taken away from their mothers (see, for example, Ballenger, 1988; Hinde and Spencer-Booth, 1971; Kaufman and Rosenblum, 1967; McKinney, 1988; Spencer-Booth and Hinde, 1967, 1971b; Suomi, et al., 1973). The latter may respond to pharmacologic agents used to treat human depression (Hrdina, et al., 1979). The infantile response to loss of an attachment figure is apparently prototypical; other losses elicit it at later stages of life.

Obviously, transient grief and depression are perfectly normal responses to severe losses. However, there are certain conditions in which loss responses appear in deviant settings. For example, chronic mourners remain severely depressed long after others would have largely recovered from an equivalent loss. Depressives become severely depressed with no obvious stimulus, or following a loss that is not commonly felt to be a major blow. In this section I review various studies which indicate that adults prone to become chronic mourners or to develop depression without a major loss differ from other persons in showing excessively salient attachment-seeking behaviors. Excessively salient childlike attachment behaviors may play a causal role in chronic mourning or depression, or may just indicate susceptibility to these disorders.

To begin with, individuals likely to develop chronic mourning tend to be dependent, especially on those they have lost, and to be generally angry (Bowlby, 1980; Parkes and Weiss, 1983). Some chronic mourners, as Bowlby (1980) observed, hide their dependency behind an aloof facade. Their anger seems to be kindled by another person's failure to meet their needs, or by insufficient enthusiasm in meeting them. Bowlby (1973) noted that children show intense anger when threatened with desertion or parental neglect or disinterest. Certain children—especially those with emotionally cold mothers—become angry following brief separations in the Ainsworth Strange Situation Test (Ainsworth, et al., 1978; Main and Weston, 1982). In a previous section, parent-child conflicts concerning parental aid were described. Children are frequently angry at parents with whom they have these conflicts, when the parents are seen as depriving them. Freud (1916), of course, considered anger toward the lost love object essential to the dynamics of pathologic mourning.

Arieti and Bemporad (1978, 1980) have described the personality type susceptible to depression. Features of their portrait agree with observations made by other observers (see, for example, Blatt, 1974; Blatt and Schichman, 1983; Blatt, et al., 1982; Bowlby, 1977, 1980; Chodoff, 1972; Matussek and Luks, 1981; Pilkonis, 1988) and with empirical studies (see, for example, Docherty, et al., 1986; Greenberg and Bornstein, 1988; Hirschfeld, et al., 1983; Matussek and Feil, 1983; Pfohl, et al., 1984; Pilkonis and Frank, 1988; Shea, et al., 1987; Smith, et al., 1988), and resemble Bowlby's (1980) description of pathological mourners. According to Arieti and Bemporad, the "predepressed" individual is unusually driven to seek love and approval. He tries to please everyone, or at least a specific person to whom he assigns a parental role. He pursues lofty goals he believes will make him lovable. Although he is often dependent, he tries to make himself useful so that others will need him.

Like chronic mourners, persons prone to depression are often very angry at the very persons from whom they seek love and approval (for discussions of the role of hostility in depression, see Abraham, 1927; Freud, 1916; Gershon, et al., 1968; Overall, et al., 1966; Pilowsky and Spence, 1975; Weissman, et al., 1971).

Most depressions are triggered by adverse events in the patients' lives (see, for example, Bebbington, et al., 1988; Brown and Harris, 1978; Lehmann, 1985; Surtees, et al., 1986; Vadher and Ndetei, 1981). Although many of these are minor by objective standards, they may have special significance for persons prone to depression. According to Arieti and Bemporad (1978, 1980), depression tends to occur when the predepressed personality type feels loss of support from a "dominant other." The dominant other is someone he has assigned a parental role. The dominant other resembles an attachment figure like those described by Bowlby (1969), but transmogrified by adult life. Loss of support may be due to death, but is more likely to be the result of divorce, desertion, family moves, withdrawal, or disagreement. The more subtle the change in the relationship to the dominant other, the more likely the change will be missed. If the change is missed, the patient may be thought to have a spontaneous illness.

Failure to reach a "dominant goal" may also lead to depression (Arieti and Bemporad, 1978, 1980). The predepressed person hopes that his dominant goal—to become rich or famous, or reach a high position—will make him more lovable to those he is trying to please. If he fails to reach a dominant goal the predepressed individual believes that he is worthless. Along the same lines, Miller (1981) describes patients who repeatedly make grandiose plans apparently intended to please an attachment figure. After each plan fails, the patients become depressed for a while.

Consistent with the hypothesis that they show excessively salient attachment-related behaviors, depressives often report chronic symptoms of panic and agoraphobia (Boyd, et al., 1984; Breier, et al., 1985; Fawcett and Kravitz, 1983; Grunhaus, 1988; Lesser, et al., 1988; Norton, et al., 1986). As I noted in the previous section, agoraphobic anxiety resembles separation and stranger anxieties normally seen in childhood, which subserve attachment relationships.

Individuals who are genetically vulnerable to depression appear to be at greater risk for pathological mourning (Raphael, 1983). I have already observed that depression runs in families with anxiety disorders, borderline personality, and other syndromes referable to dysfunction of attachment strategies (see below). Children of depressives inhibit their behavior in unfamiliar settings (Rosenbaum, et al., 1988). As I noted previously, behavioral inhibition is thought to be a measure of separation anxiety. However, behavioral abnormalities in children of depressives may be due to environmental factors, such as decreased parental responsiveness (see above), rather than to genes.

Clinicians treating pathological mourners cite a high incidence of problems in early attachment relationships (Freud, 1916; Bowlby, 1980; Volkan, 1970). Parental loss, threats of abandonment, withdrawal, neglect, or disinterest are said to be common childhood experiences among pathological mourners. Further studies are needed to verify these impressions. Bowlby (1980) cites particular beliefs—inculcated in early family relationships—predisposing to chronic grief: The belief that attachment figures are above criticism, that they must be cared for, that one is to blame should anything happen to them. Agoraphobics are said to share similar deep convictions. In spite of positive findings, studies have failed to prove that there are characteristic problems in early attachment relationships of depressed patients (see, for example, Akiskal and McKinney, 1975; Birtchnell, 1988; Brown and Harris, 1978; Crook and Eliot, 1980; Gotlib, et al., 1988; Lloyd, 1980; Parker, 1979b, 1981, 1983; Pfohl, et al., 1983; Rosenthal, et al., 1981; Rutter, 1972; Tennant, et al., 1980, 1981). This is similar to the situation noted in studies of agoraphobia (see above). It may be that early experiences increase the risk of depression only if later stresses chronically serve to elicit care-seeking behaviors. For example, Brown and his co-workers (see Brown, 1982) have shown that early parental loss predicts later problems mainly in lower class subjects, who are presumably subject to more everyday stressors. In the same vein, early loss of the mother predicts later problems in women who have had premarital pregnancies, whose lives may have thereby taken a more stressful course (Brown, 1982). Consistent with this hypothesis, maternally deprived nonhuman primates may display care-seeking behavior only after exposure to significant stressors (Hinde and Spencer-Booth, 1971; Spencer-Booth and Hinde, 1971a; Young, et al., 1973).

Like agoraphobics, and consistent with their salient attachment behaviors, chronic mourners and depressives lack self-efficacy. Cognitive therapists argue that negative expectations, especially those related to lack of personal efficacy, cause depressive disorders, and are not merely manifestations (see, for example, Abramson, et al., 1978, 1989; Bandura, 1977; Bandura, et al., 1977; Beck, 1972; Beck, et al., 1974; Costello, 1978; Ellis, 1962; Ellis and Grieger, 1977; Rizley, 1978; Seligman, 1975; Weintraub, et al., 1974; cf. Dweck and Leggett, 1988). Therapists from this school attempt to treat depression, and correct depressive tendencies, by altering beliefs related to personal efficacy. McKinney (1988) reviews animal studies pertinent to these cognitive models of affective illness.

The individual who feels inefficacious, and in particular feels incapable of competing with others, tends to be submissive. Competitive behaviors are discussed in the following chapter. Suffice it to say here that submissive behavior patterns skirt interpersonal conflict by yielding claims for resources which otherwise might be fought for. As one would expect of individuals who underestimate self-efficacy or RHP, and who have an exaggerated need for approval, depressed patients are inappropriately submissive in conflictual situations. By decreasing reinforcement, lack of assertiveness may even worsen depression. This is one rationale for treating depression with assertiveness training (see, for example, Lazarus, 1971, 1974; Lazarus and Serber, 1968; Lewinsohn and Shaffer, 1971; Libet and Lewinsohn, 1973). A number of authors (see, for example, Lewis, 1934; Price, 1967, 1969, 1972; Price and Sloman, 1984; Sloman, 1981, 1983; Sloman, et al., 1979) have proposed viewing depression as a form of submissive behavior triggered by perceived defeat in the social arena. The model espoused here differs from the "submissiveness" model by emphasizing what the depressive does do—he seeks approval and nurturance—rather than what he doesn't do: he doesn't assert himself.

Borderline Personality

Numerous studies have now clarified the picture of borderline personality (see, for example, Barrash, et al., 1983; Clarkin, et al., 1983; Grinker, 1979; Gunderson and Kolb, 1978; Gunderson, et al., 1975; Koenigsberg, et al., 1983; Kroll, et al., 1981; McGlashan, 1983a, 1983b; Perry and Klerman, 1980; Pope, et al., 1983; Sheehy, et al., 1980; Soloff and Ulrich, 1981; Spitzer, et al., 1979). In this section I will show how symptoms and signs of borderline personality, together with certain etiologic factors, can be rendered intelligible by placing them in relation to childhood strategies aimed at obtaining aid. Looked at from this vantage point, the borderline patient is much like the patient susceptible to chronic mourning or depression, but more severely disturbed, with more deviant manifestations of childhood social strategies.

First, like other patients described in this chapter, borderline patients are frequently dependent and angry. Relationships formed by borderlines differ from those formed by agoraphobics and depressives in that the care-seeking element is more obvious and childlike, and in that anger, being poorly controlled, plays a more prominent role. Typical borderline patients may be so angered by minor disappointments from other people who serve as attachment figures that they cannot sustain relationships. These end repeatedly on an acrimonious note (cf. Adler, 1979 on therapeutic relationships; cf. Akhtar and Byrne, 1983; Kernberg, 1975; Volkan, 1976 on "splitting" into good and bad representations). Fear of domination by attachment figures may add to the instability of borderline interactions (Melges and Swartz, 1989).

Borderline patients are anxious when separated from persons on whom they feel dependent. Typically, their anxiety takes the severe form seen in agoraphobia and depressive disorders. To explain this severe separation anxiety, various authors have argued that borderlines lack "object constancy" (see, for example, Blanck and Blanck, 1974). "Object constancy" is a term borrowed from Piaget, who used it to denote an unrelated phenomenon (see Hartmann, 1952, 1953; Piaget, 1954; Bower, 1974). Its use in connection with borderlines only leads to confusion.

Borderline patients are also prone to become depressed following minor losses (see, for example, Akiskal, 1981; Bell, et al., 1983; Carroll, et al., 1981; Charney, et al., 1981; Garbutt, et al., 1983; Liebowitz and Klein, 1981; McGlashan, 1983a, 1983b; Pope, et al., 1983; Soloff, et al., 1982). In the previous section, I argued that individuals prone to develop depression differ from other persons by virtue of excessively salient childlike attachment behaviors.

Borderline patients are often alcohol, sedative, or narcotic abusers. In the psychoanalytic literature, drug addiction has been treated as an "oral" trait, implying a link to early attachment relationships (see Fenichel, 1945). Pharmacologic studies show that opiates, at least, alleviate infantile separation distress akin to what I hypothesize is felt by borderline patients (see below).

Sexual promiscuity, perversions, and gender confusion are common in borderline patients. Of course, human sexual life is more complex than the sexual life of any other species. Nonetheless, sexual dysfunctions shown by borderline patients resemble sexual deviations shown by nonhuman primates deprived of early maternal care (Goldfoot, 1977; Harlow, 1971; Mason, 1963; Mitchell, 1968, 1970).

Finally, borderline patients may harm themselves when angry, depressed, or anxious. Self-mutilation may occur following the breakdown of an important relationship, or when the patient is angry at someone on whom he or she depends. Nonhuman primates raised without attachment figures also mutilate themselves when they are made angry or anxious (Brandt, et al., 1971; Mason, et al., 1968). Primate self-mutilation has sometimes been considered a self-directed manifestation of generalized hyperaggression seen in primates deprived of early care (Arling and Harlow, 1967; Gluck and Sackett, 1974; Goldfoot, 1977; Harlow and Harlow, 1965; Mason, 1963; Mitchell, 1968, 1970; Pugh, 1977; Salzen, 1979).

I have already noted that borderline personality runs in families with anxiety syndromes, depression, and other disorders referable to dysfunction of attachment strategies, or of the psychological mechanisms subserving them. Consistent with the notion that borderline personality is an attachment disorder, and with the prominence of symptoms—such as sexual abnormalities and self-mutilation— seen in primate models of attachment deprivation, there appears to be strong evidence that many borderline patients have suffered disruptions in early attachment relationships. Very early maternal separations, deviant parenting styles, coldness, neglect, and severe abuse have all been shown to be common in the histories of patients with borderline personality or with features of borderline personality (Bradley, 1979; Bryer, 1987; Gunderson, et al., 1980; Herman, 1986; Herman, et al., 1989; Johansen, 1983; Lindemann, 1960; Sheldon, 1988; Stone, 1981). Mahler (1971) argued that borderline personality results from miscarriage of the separation-individuation process in the second year of life. As I noted earlier, the separation-individuation process described by Mahler and her co-workers (1975) may represent a stage in the evolution of parent-child conflicts, which are exacerbated by the child's increasing motor capacities. A recently developed cognitive approach to borderline personality emphasizes deficits in various coping skills, which are said to be due to parents who are unwilling to tolerate expression of negative affects (Linehan, 1987; Swenson, 1989).

Other Syndromes

Certain important syndromes seem to be linked to depression. Chronic pain syndromes (Blumer and Heilbronn, 1981; Kramlinger, et al., 1983), obsessive-compulsive disease (Capstick, 1971; Coryell,

1981; Insel and Murphy, 1981; Rasmussen and Tsuang, 1986), post-traumatic stress disorder (Bleich, et al., 1986; Falcon, et al., 1985; Hogben and Cornfield, 1981; Horowitz, et al., 1980), somatization disorder (Coryell and Norten, 1981), and bulimia (Hudson, et al., 1982, 1983; Levy, et al., 1989; Mitchell, et al., 1985; Swift, et al., 1986) overlap with depressive illness genetically, phenomenologically, or pharmacologically. Insofar as these disorders represent variants of depressive illness, the model developed here predicts that those prone to develop them will show excessively salient childlike attachment aims.

As I noted above, opiates inhibit separation distress shown by nonhuman infants (Fabre-Nys, et al., 1982; Panksepp, et al., 1978; Pettijohn, 1979; Pettijohn, et al., 1977). This suggests that individuals with excessively salient attachment-related behaviors or psychological processes might be at increased risk to become opiate addicts. Consistent with this suggestion, depressive disorders are common among opiate addicts (Rounsaville, et al., 1982). Along the same lines, alcoholism is common in families of patients with depression and panic disorder (Reich, 1988), which suggests that alcohol may also be used to treat dysphoric states subserving attachment strategies (see Keller, 1988).

Fisher and Greenberg (1985) review the evidence concerning the existence of an "oral" character type. Individuals showing this particular character type are dependent, submissive, and fearful of rejection. I noted above that dependent and aid-seeking behaviors, which are prominent features of the oral character type, are common in patients with agoraphobic, depressive, or borderline symptoms.

In the following chapter I discuss Draper and Harpending's (1988) model of hysteria. Childlike attachment-seeking behaviors may play a greater role in the genesis of hysteria than Draper and Harpending indicate.

Not surprisingly, in light of the role of anger in childhood social strategies, unfortunate early attachment events are also at the root of certain aggressive disorders. For example, it is now well established that child abusers are very likely to have been victims of child abuse themselves (DeLozier, 1982; Zeanah and Zeanah, 1989). Kuhn's (1958) case history of a patient called "Rudolph" shows how murderous feelings toward women may also result from early attachment losses. Rudolph's violent behavior resembles the type of aggression shown by borderline patients.

Finally, there is the problem of manic-depressive disorder. Depressive episodes experienced by manic-depressive patients are essentially indistinguishable from episodes of depression experienced by unipolar depressives (Brockington, et al., 1982; Abrams and Taylor, 1974, 1980). Like the latter, they resemble prototypical loss responses shown by children in response to attachment disruptions. Manic-depressives, however, also experience other abnormal mental states, which, like depression, often develop in response to losses (see Lehmann, 1985). When in these other states, which are categorized together as forms or stages of mania (see Carlson and Goodwin, 1973; Kraepelin, 1921), manic-depressives may be euphoric, hyperactive, agitated, or disorganized, and may experience delusions or hallucinations appropriate to their mood. Psychotic symptoms are discussed in the following chapter. Patients in so-called mixed states experience elements of the depressive syndrome together with elements of a manic presentation.

The variety of mental states considered to be forms or stages of mania precludes any simple analysis in ethological terms. For example, observing that mania is triggered by the same types of loss that trigger depression, psychoanalysts argued that it is a defense (Fenichel, 1945; Freud, 1916; Lewin, 1932). According to this view, the manic denies his depression by assuming an opposite attitude. Sociobiologically, this would suggest that manic-depressives are similar to depressives, but alter their loss responses through psychological processes. However, this view cannot account for other elements of manic presentations, such as agitation, fearfulness, and disorganization. Likewise, Gardner (1982) considered mania an abnormal dominance state opposite to the submissive states seen in depressive illness (see above). In his euphoric, expansive stage the manic-depressive exudes dominance signals inappropriate to his real social condition. He seems to experience delusionally high subjective RHP, self-esteem, and self-efficacy, and his behavior is concomitantly aggressive and domineering. Gardner's view, however, is more a description of one aspect of mania than a general theory of manic states, since these can take other forms or change from day to day.

What may be common to all the states subsumed under the rubric of mania is intense psychological and behavioral excitation, which stands in contrast to the usual inhibition seen in manic–depressives when they are depressed (cf. Lehmann, 1985). If this is so, the manic-depressive is like the unipolar depressive in his sensitivity to loss and in his propensity toward apparently spontaneous shifts in state, but whereas the abnormal mental state in the unipolar depressive takes a prototypical, inhibited, form, it can take on excited forms in the manic-depressive. This view could account for the fact that psychostimulants or activating antidepressants can precipitate manic states when used to treat retarded bipolar depressions (Davis and Sharma, 1986; Goodwin and Roy-Byrne, 1987; Potter, et al., 1987; Wehr, et al., 1987).

According to Nesse's (1989) Resource Allocation Model, normal high and low mood states are associated with biases respectively promoting or inhibiting resource allocations. Elevated mood states predispose individuals to risk their resources on uncertain ventures, whereas depressed mood states predispose individuals to conserve their resources. If viewed in Nesse's terms, pathological mood states consequent on losses can be seen as alternative tactics for dealing with serious setbacks, taken to their extremes. The depressive, inhibited response corresponds to a tactic of resource conservation, or hunkering down. In depression, however, the hunkering down is exaggerated so that it becomes dysfunctional. Euphoric, excited responses correspond to a tactic of increased investment, or making up for the loss by dint of increased activity. In manic states, however, the increased activity is frantic and degenerates into senselessness, and the new investments, insofar as they can be discerned, are unrealistic.

In a previous section, I argued that individuals sensitive to losses tend to be characterized by excessively salient attachment-related behaviors. Insofar as manic-depressives show the same sensitivity to losses as depressives, but differ in being able to enter excited, as well as inhibited states, they too might show care-seeking behaviors resembling those of the child. Too little data exists on the personalities of manic-depressive patients to really address this hypothesis. Arieti and Bemporad (1978) and other authors (Chodoff, 1972; Cohen, et al., 1954) have identified personality traits characteristic of manic-depressives that are similar to those of depressives and that point toward salient attachment-related dynamics. However, many manic-depressives, who are said to be "cyclothymic," demonstrate large fluctuations in their energy and activity levels (Akiskal, et al., 1977). These fluctuations dominate everyday functioning and obscure what might otherwise be more recognizable patterns.

Manic-depressive illness is known to be strongly determined by genetic factors, which apparently partly coincide with genetic factors producing depressive illness (see, for example, Baron, et al., 1981; Clayton, 1981; Coryell, et al., 1984; Gershon, et al., 1975; Goldin and Gershon, 1988; Jakimow-Venulet, 1981; Sperber and Jarvik, 1976; Tsuang, et al., 1985; Weissman, Gershon, et al., 1984; Winokur, 1980; Winokur, et al., 1982). Children of manic-depressives exhibit behavioral problems (Decina, et al., 1983; Gershon, et al., 1985), but these may not be referable to problems with attachment, or may result from environmental factors. Very little is known about the early attachment experiences of manic-depressives. However, since parents of manic-depressives frequently turn out to have been alcoholic or mentally ill (see above references), many manic-depressives no doubt experienced difficult early relationships.

4

Relationships with Adults

I n this chapter I will discuss some innately probable strategies evident in relationships between adults. Kin altruism, which I discussed in earlier chapters and which is so important in parent-child relations, will not be dealt with here. Although kin altruism affects kinship systems and social mores, and hence is important in relationships between adults, heuristic clarity dictates that attention be directed here toward other social strategies. These social strategies are salient in relationships between unrelated or distantly related adults, for whom kin altruism would be a minor factor. Kin altruism can be treated as an additional factor complicating these strategies when genetic kinship becomes a significant matter.

The most obvious fact about adults is that they live their lives in stable social groups composed of other adults and dependent children. Two social strategies entail affiliation with a group and with its members. In the sociobiologic literature, these have been called "mutualism" (Wrangham, 1982) and "reciprocal altruism" (Trivers, 1971). Mutualism is equivalent or related to "synergistic selection" (Maynard Smith, 1982), "weak altruism" (Wilson, 1979, 1980), and "indirect reciprocity" (Alexander, 1987), among other terms. Though mutualism and reciprocal altruism are closely related strategies, reciprocity being a special form of cooperation (see, for example, Krebs, 1987), they require different social skills for their realization. I will therefore discuss them separately.

Mutualism

Mutualism, as I am using the term, refers to a social strategy. Individuals adhering to this strategy cooperate with others whenever possible to achieve common, or mutually beneficial, goals. These goals are not achievable, or are achieved less efficiently, through individual action. By beneficial, I refer to inclusive fitness. "Whenever possible" is an important qualification. Many species carry out isolated cooperative acts while lacking a general tendency toward cooperative efforts (see, for example, Buskirk, 1975; Lin and Michener, 1972; West-Eberhard, 1978). The cooperative acts in these cases do not seem to manifest a general social strategy. There are species of spiders, for instance, who jointly spin their webs. But spiders of these species apparently cannot cooperate for purposes other than spinning. These spiders, so to speak, can perform a particular minuet, but they cannot waltz or square dance. They lack the impulse to dance together other than in their minuet. By contrast, humans and some nonhuman primates, especially chimpanzees (see, for example, Itani and Suzuki, 1967; Lawick-Goodall, 1968, 1971; Sugiyama, 1969; Suzuki, 1971; Teleki, 1973), cooperate with each other to achieve whatever goals are important at the moment. These goals, together with the steps needed to reach them, are only partly predictable. Individuals learn new roles; they do whatever is needed to further the common endeavor. Some primates can really be said to adhere to a social strategy, embodied in varied efforts carried out with others.

Group life offers advantages even without the benefits conferred by mutualism. For example, ecological models show that just being near to others decreases the chance that a given individual will fall victim to predators (Hamilton, 1971). Predation has been an important force in primate evolution (see Alexander, et al., 1979). Proximity to others permits adaptive learning. Even nonhuman primate groups can acquire simple practices and technologies, which are then used by their members (Itani and Nishimura, 1973; Kawai, 1965; Lawick-Goodall, 1968, 1971; Tsumori, 1967). Every human group has a subsistence technology far too complex to be discovered anew by smaller social aggregates.

With mutualism, however, the advantages of group life are greatly amplified. For example, members of nonhuman primate groups need not rely on just being near to others to reduce their risk of predation. Instead they cooperate to mount active defenses against their natural predators (Altmann and Altmann, 1970; Hall, 1960;

Schaller, 1963; Washburn and DeVore, 1961). Protohominid groups, which occupied an ecological niche like that of modern baboons, no doubt defended themselves against very similar dangers. As the threat of predation waned, hominid group defenses were likely employed against other bands (Alexander, 1979, 1987; Alexander, et al., 1979). Modern-day primitive human groups face little threat of predation but cooperate to defend themselves against other human beings. To mention another example, groups of chimpanzees also hunt together in cooperative fashion (Lawick-Goodall, 1968, 1971; Suzuki, 1971; Teleki, 1973). By coordinating their actions, chimpanzee hunting groups bring down prey which a single individual would be unable to kill. The range and size of prey possible for a hunting group is increased disproportionately to the pooled caloric needs of the individual members. Organized hominid bands were able to kill the largest animals of their time (Fox, 1980; Mellen, 1981).

If there are inclusive fitness benefits achievable through mutualism, and if these are limited to those who help achieve them, then mutualism is evolutionarily stable. Cooperative individuals will always be better off than those disinclined to cooperate. The latter lose the advantages of coordinated activities. Also, many cooperative activities harm individuals who are not taking part (Wrangham, 1982). For instance, predators thwarted by groups turn their attention to loners. Cooperative groups can also monopolize food supplies, leaving those who go it alone without adequate sustenance. In cases like these, nonparticipants not only gain none of the benefits of cooperation, they suffer other losses because they have gone it alone.

If the benefits of cooperation are available to those who do not actually help to achieve them, mutualism will suffer. In this case, the best strategy will be to avoid doing one's share. For example, an individual protected by coordinated group defense would have an advantage if he could avoid taking part in it. An individual sharing the catch would have an advantage if he could avoid the hunting. Since the gain to the shirker is frequently a loss to those who cooperate, individuals who cooperate with each other must insure that benefits flow only to those who really help to achieve them. At the least they must be wary of those who do not participate in their mutual ventures.

Essentially all human beings live or have lived in social groups organized in part for mutualistic purposes. The few exceptions are considered below. Pre-agrarian human groups ranged in size from a few dozen to two or three hundred persons (Lenski, 1970; cf. Festinger, 1986). Groups larger than these were probably unable to coordinate their activities without hierarchical structures. Common activities included hunting and defense. Modern-day hunter-gatherer groups that grow excessively large fission into smaller groups that go their separate ways (Chagnon, 1979b). When such groups divide, they do so in such a way as to increase in-group relatedness (Chagnon, 1979b; cf. Chepko-Sade, 1979). Consequently, groups are composed of persons more or less closely related. Obviously, kin–altruistic tendencies promote in-group harmony (cf. Maynard Smith, 1964, 1976b; Michod, 1982 on the interrelation of group process and kin altruism). Population densities increase with agrarianism (Lenski, 1970); people no longer have contact with all members of their group. But greater productivity from agrarianism supports a ruling class that coordinates endeavors on a larger scale (see Schmookler, 1984). These endeavors have been, unfortunately, mostly related to warfare. Societies have world views to justify their rulers (Berger and Luckmann, 1966). Even in larger societies, though, smaller groups usually form whenever needs arise that require cooperation on a more limited scale. People may go so far as to identify with these groups in place of the larger collective (see, for example, Sherif, 1966; Tajfel, 1974, 1978, 1979).

Being universal and evolutionarily stable, mutualism is an innately probable strategy in the sense described in chapter 2.

Innate Dispositions Promoting Mutualism

Several ubiquitous dispositions promote adherence to mutualism. Though these dispositions, like many others, might be successfully combatted by systematic training, or environmental manipulation, their universality indicates they are readily acquired. Traits are readily acquired if they are somehow more consistent with innate characteristics determining epigenesis than are alternative traits (see Lumsden and Wilson, 1981, 1983). All of the dispositions described below depend on social perceptions, communicational skills, and affective responses known to be dependent on limbic, language, and other centers in the nervous system. Biologic factors—genetic and extragenetic—can alter some of the dispositions under discussion here (see below).

The first disposition promoting mutualism is a propensity to categorize other persons as in-group members or nonmembers, depending upon whether they belong to the same cooperative group. The group may be anything from a tribe to a trade union. Since members of the group cooperate with each other, but not necessarily with nonmembers, the in-group, out-group distinction is usually an invidious one. In general, the more encompassing the group, the more invidious the distinction is likely to be in practice. Uncooperative, hostile feelings, if they are expressed, are much more often directed outside the group.

Invidious in-group distinctions, sometimes manifested in violence, are found in cultures with widely disparate political and economic systems (see, for example, Berger and Luckmann, 1966; Campbell, 1978; Divale and Harris, 1976; Durham, 1976; Ember, 1978; Erikson, 1968, 1969; Lorenz, 1960; Lumsden and Wilson, 1981; Tiger, 1984; Tiger and Fox, 1971; Wilson, 1975). Therefore, though they are mobilized for political and economic functions, invidious in-group distinctions are not the result of those systems. In fact, laboratory studies show that invidious in-group distinctions are readily elicited with artificial groups lacking definite interests of any kind whatsoever (Billig and Tajfel, 1973; Brewer and Silver, 1978; Tajfel, 1970, 1981, 1982; Tajfel and Billig, 1974). Schmookler (1984) argues successfully, though, that postagrarian cultures have been selected-for according to their effectiveness in prosecuting hostilities toward other groups. Insofar as Schmookler is right, cultural selection has favored social arrangements which cultivate and exaggerate pre-existing dispositions promoting external hostility.

Psychological processes akin to "identification" (see below) may promote invidious in-group distinctions.

Second, threatened or real alienation from a social group produces affective distress. Affective distress is a negative reinforcer promoting cooperation. For example, some primitive tribes excommunicate persons who have violated taboos (see Cannon, 1942). The ensuing affective upheaval oftentimes proves lethal. Galanter

(1978, 1989) called attention to milder forms of the same type of distress occurring in modern societies. According to Galanter, disaffiliated individuals suffer neurotic symptoms. They gravitate to small groups such as religious cults, which have a beneficial effect by providing a sense of belonging. In Galanter's (1978) study, relief of neurotic distress consequent on membership in a religious cult correlated most highly with stated distrust of outsiders. Bellah and his colleagues (1985) have shown how difficult it is to achieve a sense of belonging in modern American society. Some of the factors they cite are common to all developed societies. I have elsewhere reviewed the evidence in favor of Galanter's theory (Wenegrat, 1989). Both cult phenomena and more mundane religious beliefs can be partly accounted for by relief of affective distress consequent on membership in a cohesive group (see below).

Finally, persons everywhere conform to the world view characteristic of their group (see, for example, Berger and Luckmann, 1966; Durkheim, 1965; Pareto, 1963). Cognitive conformity promotes solidarity and unified action. Conformity results in part from early acculturation. However, laboratory studies have shown that beliefs are also determined by current social cues (Asch, 1956; Crutchfield, 1955; Jacobs and Campbell, 1961; Sherif, 1937). This may be especially true for social and ethical mores (see, for example, Milgram, 1965, 1974). As expected from the sociobiological model, more closely knit experimental groups are able to elicit greater degrees of conformity (Berkowitz, 1954; Sakurai, 1975).

Although certain cultures, at certain times, seem to discourage conformity, laboratory studies show that some tendency to conform is ubiquitous (Milgram, 1961; Nicholson, et al., 1985; Whittaker and Meade, 1967).

Ideologic and religious conversions demonstrate the effectiveness of group cognitive models. Most men and women adopt rather uncritically whatever ideology is espoused by their social group. For this reason, successful religious or ideologic recruitment proceeds by making the convert feel part of a group. Once this has been achieved, ideology or theology follow without much effort (see, Wenegrat, 1989).

Like invidious feelings toward outsiders, tendencies toward conformity are exploited for political and economic ends. Conformity is especially used in preparing for organized warfare. Schmookler's thesis (see above), consequently, is as relevant to conformity as to invidious feelings directed outside the group.

Reciprocal Altruism

In chapter 2 I described kin directed altruism. Parental aid and proximity maintenance, described in chapter 3, are forms of kin altruism. But kin altruism is only part of the story. Altruistic behaviors are often directed toward non-kin, or toward kin too distantly related to justify the costs of altruistic actions. Altruistic behaviors are even seen directed toward other species (see Trivers, 1971).

It is important that the reader recall the distinction drawn in chapter 2 between the uses of "altruism." The commonsense use of this term implies intentionality. The biologic use implies no conscious intention, or even any awareness of the act itself.

Reciprocal altruism is a social strategy that helps to account for altruistic behaviors directed toward non-kin (see Trivers, 1971). A reciprocal altruist will provide cost-efficient aid to anyone who needs it, unless the potential beneficiary is known to be unwilling to provide the same type of aid. The unwilling individual is known to be unwilling on the basis of past refusals. By cost-efficient, I refer to aid that is important to the recipient but not terribly costly to the altruist. Throwing a rope to a person drowning in a lake is highly cost-efficient. Jumping in may be less so.

In a group composed mostly of reciprocal altruists, reciprocal altruism is highly advantageous and evolutionarily stable. A reciprocal altruist living with other reciprocal altruists can expect to do numerous favors that cost him rather little, and to receive many favors, some of which are important. He may have to throw many ropes, so to speak, but one may be thrown to him. The one thrown to him will outweigh, in inclusive fitness terms, all those he has had to throw. On the other hand, individuals in such a group who deviate from the reciprocal altruism strategy, by indiscriminate generosity or by selfishness, will be penalized. Indiscriminate altruists aid unrelated individuals who are unlikely to reciprocate, should the occasion arise. They also reduce the incentive for altruism in general. Consequently, in comparison with reciprocal altruists, they wind up giving more aid for the amount they receive. Selfish individuals save themselves the cost of aiding others, but lose the greater benefits of aid from reciprocal altruists. To the extent that aiding others is in fact cost-efficient, selfishness leads to a loss.

Actually, as long as the cost of altruism is modest, reciprocal altruists, as I have defined them, do well in comparison with numerous other strategists, almost without regard to whether or not they are common. Axelrod (1984; see also Axelrod and Hamilton, 1981) studied strategies for the Prisoner's Dilemma, a two person game formally resembling the situation existing between a reciprocal altruist and his or her potential beneficiary. The Prisoner's Dilemma has been extensively researched by mathematical theorists (see, for example, Davis, 1983; Owen, 1982; Shubik, 1982). Computerized iterations of the Prisoner's Dilemma, pitting various strategies against one another, showed that a strategy called Tit-for-Tat was the most robust and successful in spite of initial conditions. Players adhering to Tit-for-Tat cooperate with another player unless that other player betrayed them on the preceding round. Tit-for-Tat resembles reciprocal altruism with the most optimistic assumption, consistent with reciprocal altruism, about the other's intentions.

Humans in every society act like reciprocal altruists (see Gouldner, 1960; cf. Mauss, 1954). They frequently proffer aid to familiar persons who are not necessarily kin. More cost-effective aid, being more vital to the recipient and less costly to the altruist, is provided most readily. And if cost-effective aid is withheld, it is probably because the potential beneficiary has withheld similar aid on previous occasions. Like mutualism, reciprocal altruism is therefore innately probable in the sense described in chapter 2.

Innate Dispositions Promoting
Reciprocal Altruism

Certain cognitive and affective dispositions lead men and women to be reciprocal altruists. Though they may be affected by systematic training or environmental manipulation, at the very least these dispositions are readily acquired in disparate cultural settings. As I noted above, in relation to dispositions promoting adherence to mutualism, ease of acquisition implies a certain consistency with biological factors reflecting human genes. As with mutualism, the dispositions promoting reciprocal altruism involve perceptual, communicative, and affective processes dependent on brain structures, and biological processes can alter these dispositions (see below).

To adhere to reciprocal altruism, individuals must live in stable groups. In a stable group, altruists can learn something about potential beneficiaries. There are opportunities to provide appropriate aid to those who are altruistic. Isolated individuals, who have only fleeting encounters with other individuals, may be altruistic or not but they cannot be truly contingent, reciprocal altruists. Consequently, all the dispositions cited above, which promote long-term mutualistic relationships, also lay the groundwork for reciprocal altruism.

Taking leads from Sigmund Freud (1914) and Anna Freud (1966), Badcock (1986) proposed that the innate psychological basis for altruistic behaviors is "identification," the tendency to see oneself as the same as the other. As I noted earlier, identification may also explain relative in-group harmony (see Hornstein, 1978). Badcock argued that genes promote altruism via their effects on mental processes causing identification. According to Sigmund Freud (1921, 1923), identification is involved in all strong emotional bonds. Social modeling and imitative processes, which presuppose a type of identification (see Fenichel, 1945), appear to be fundamental to human social relations (see Bandura, 1986).

A number of authors have recently stressed the emotional, as opposed to cognitive, cues for altruistic behaviors (see, for example, Hoffman, 1982; MacDonald, 1988b). Brothers (1989) described the known biological substrates for emotional empathy, which has long been thought to motivate altruistic acts (see Richards, 1987). Clinically, altruistic tendencies often seem to fluctuate with affective state (Jenner, 1978). For example, some depressed patients, especially those with obsessional traits, are notably unaltruistic. Expansive hypomanics or manics, by contrast, frequently offer others aid they cannot afford to give. Mood-related changes in altruistic tendencies may be due to changes in RHP or self-efficacy which accompany affective illness (see chapter 3 and below). In effect, the depressed patient does not believe he can afford to be helpful; the expansive manic feels he can afford to give anything. I have already noted that affective states, as well as obsessional symptoms, are determined in part by factors of a biological type.

People become hostile to those who refuse them aid, especially if that aid could have been easily given. Hostility elicited by failure to offer aid insures adherence to the contingency which is part of reciprocal altruism: to refuse aid to those who have proven unwilling to offer aid themselves. The temporal course of hostility is also most likely adaptive in relation to reciprocal altruism. Hostile feelings elicited by lack of generosity most often fade with time, or when social relations take a turn for the better. Axelrod's (1984) study of the iterated Prisoner's Dilemma, which formally resembles reciprocal altruism, showed that the most successful strategies were ones that forgave opponents rather quickly after betrayals. "Grudge-holding" strategies were unable to correct an initial impression at odds with statistical averages. Limbic and temporal lobe centers apparently modulate hostile feelings in humans and other mammals (see, for example, Eichelman, 1986).

Insofar as hostility leads to aggressive behavior, it may promote altruism in the group at large. Reluctant altruists may prefer to offer aid, which is after all not too costly, than face moralistic aggression consequent on refusal.

A number of authors have noted how reciprocal altruism depends on the interplay of various social skills (see, for example, Alexander, 1987; Badcock, 1986; Trivers, 1971, 1981). For example, individuals who have not been altruistic benefit substantially if they can make their stinginess appear in a better light, or if they can persuade others that they have changed their ways. Reciprocal altruists, consequently, must be able to guard against deception, without simply shutting the door on everyone who once lapsed from altruistic behavior. Social skills required to persuade and to guard against deception are distinctively human, at least in developed form (for example, see Kummer, 1978). Highly advanced social skills of the type at issue here depend on prefrontal cortex, which is especially developed in human beings (Blumer and Benson, 1975; Hecaen and Albert, 1975; Lishman, 1987). Trivers (1971), in fact, has argued that social demands imposed by reciprocal altruism caused the rapid increase in human cerebral size during the Pleistocene epoch.

Alienation

Stable social affiliations are needed for both mutualism and reciprocal altruism. I have already noted that affective dispositions maintain affiliations and motivate formation of new affiliations when old ones are attenuated. Insofar as they are innate, these dispositions may have evolved because they promoted adherence to these advantageous strategies. External circumstances might contrive, though, to deprive individuals of old affiliations while blocking formation of new ones. Circumstances like these were probably rare throughout human prehistory. Individuals were born into and lived their lives in small groups of interrelated persons who hunted, gathered, and when necessary, fought together against other men and beasts (see Festinger, 1986). No sane person would voluntarily leave such a group, and the rare person extruded from it would probably have perished in rather short order. Cultural, economic, and historical circumstances, though, have now made once rare events common. Modern history is characterized by migration. Many individuals leave the groups in which they were raised. They may even move to where a new language is spoken. Even without migration, the dynamics of modern culture might make it more difficult to maintain affiliations with larger-than-family groups (see Bellah, et al., 1985).

Individuals without a place in a stable social group lack opportunity for mutualism or reciprocal altruism. Consequently, these strategies should be much less salient than in the behavior of persons securely embedded in social groups. To the extent they are evident at all, their manifestations might be sporadic, truncated, or dysfunctional; in the absence of strong group bonds, the social feedback processes requisite to their realization are likely to be deficient. Psychiatric disorders manifesting dysfunction of group-related strategies—mutualism and reciprocal altruism—should increase in frequency when the social milieu attenuates these strategies in their normal form (see below).

I noted above that distress due to disaffiliation from stable social groups promotes adherence to strategies contingent on group membership. I described Galanter's (1978, 1989) theory, that disaffiliation from larger-than-family groups causes neurotic distress, which may be alleviated by joining religious cults. Some of what Galanter refers to may be what people feel when they say they are "lonely." Studies show that self-reported loneliness is less a measure of isolation than of perceived exclusion from close-knit social groups (Audy, 1980; Rubenstein and Shaver, 1980; Sermat, 1980). Weiss

(1982) noted that loneliness is like "separation distress," except that it typically lacks a highly specified object. The object may be the social group and not a particular member.

Studies of so-called extrinsically or consensually religious persons (Allen and Spilka, 1967; Allport, 1966; Allport and Ross, 1967) indicate that frustrated group affiliative motives are of even more widespread importance than Galanter seems to imply. Joining cultlike groups may be just the most obvious way in which people remedy lack of affiliation. Mainstream religious or other groups may serve the very same function. Extrinsically or consensually religious persons, who comprise a large proportion of those who describe themselves as mainstream religious, tend to be ethnically and racially prejudiced, highly attuned to social rules (Hunt and King, 1971), and preoccupied with social status and categories (Pargament, et al., 1979; Spilka, 1977). Their religiosity seems to be motivated more by a desire to belong to a cohesive group than by a genuine interest in religious faith (see Wenegrat, 1989). Group-related motives tend to be neglected in the psychotherapy of religious persons.

Delusions

As I noted above, members of a social group adopt its consensual reality, at least in its basic form. Persons who are delusional, though, create their own world view based on their preoccupations, or what Wernicke (cited in Binswanger, 1958) called their "overvalent ideas." These preoccupations might be depressive, hypochondriacal, grandiose, self-referential, or persecutory, or they might take other forms, but they are invariably intense and affectively charged, even when not expressed in a delusional form. In general, delusions appear in the setting of disorders, such as depression or schizotypy, in which intense preoccupations play a prominent role.

Delusions of almost all types respond to the same medications, which are dopamine blocking agents (Creese, et al., 1976; Peroutka and Snyder, 1980). This suggests that delusions of almost all types depend on the same physiologic process. That is, there must be a common pathway through which preoccupations assume a delusional mantle, and that common pathway must involve dopamine neurons. Studies of newer agents suggest alternative neurochemical theories (see Snyder and Largent, 1989). A typical clinical finding is that when delusions are treated, the underlying preoccupations—depressive, distrustful, or schizotypal—are nonetheless still evident, but in nondelusional form. These preoccupations require additional therapy. For example, once in remission, patients with schizophrenic or paranoid disorders may benefit from treatment aimed at increasing the saliency of consensual views (see below, also Gunderson, 1979). Patients with mood disorders may need psychotherapy and also antidepressants or other medications to stabilize their mood (Arieti and Bemporad, 1978). I have elsewhere suggested that delusions and certain other psychotic symptoms are akin to fever (Wenegrat, 1984). Fever occurs in many somatic illnesses but may take a characteristic form in one or another disorder. The same agents can be used to treat fever, regardless of the illness in which it has supervened, but treating the fever does not cure the disorder.

Apparently, dopamine blocking agents exert their antipsychotic effects, including their effects on delusions, by blocking neurotransmission from meso-cortical and meso-limbic dopamine tracts (Davidson, et al., 1986; Watson, et al., 1986). The meso-cortical tract terminates in the frontal lobe. I have already noted that frontal lobe activity appears to regulate complex social behaviors. Chronically psychotic schizophrenic patients manifest social deficits, deficits in their thinking, and physiologic abnormalities plausibly indicative of frontal lobe dysfunction (Berman, et al., 1988; Goldberg, et al., 1987; Weinberger and Kleinman, 1986; Weinberger, et al., 1988). The meso-limbic tract terminates on limbic structures that appear to regulate affect. Meso-cortical and meso-limbic activity must somehow affect the relative salience of private preoccupations, consensual constructs, and current social cues. It is especially interesting in this regard that nonconsensual, idiosyncratic preoccupations expressed by schizotypes who are not acutely psychotic may also diminish with dopamine blockers (see Schulz, et al., 1988).

Schizotypal Personality

Schizoid individuals are socially isolative (American Psychiatric Association, 1987). Their tendency to withdraw is established early in life, often in adolescence, and becomes a lifelong pattern. Though they may enjoy being with members of their family of origin, they otherwise prefer to be by themselves. They may be emotionally cold and pervasively lacking in empathy, and they are often fearful of others. They usually do not marry. Many schizoids find occupations that allow them to work alone, but the most severely disturbed of them fail to earn a living.

Schizotypal individuals are also isolative. In addition, though, their thinking is inconsistent with their cultural norms (American Psychiatric Association, 1987). They tend to have highly autistic philosophic, religious, or magical ideas, which cannot be understood by normal persons. The term "autistic," which is frequently used in relation to schizotypal ideas, implies an endogenous, as opposed to external origin (see Hinsie and Campbell, 1970). Schizotypal responses to psychological tests—especially projective tests— are also hard to follow (Gilbert, 1980; Rapaport, et al., 1968). These responses tend to be at least statistically deviant; they are offered without much effort to render them more comprehensible.

Schizoid and schizotypal personality disorders are related to schizophrenia: First, all three diagnoses are characterized by withdrawal and by some degree of idiosyncracy. Schizoid persons are the least idiosyncratic. Schizotypal persons have autistic preoccupations; schizophrenics express these preoccupations in delusional form (see Siever and Klar, 1986). Second, schizoid and schizotypal personality disorders are genetically inherited alongside schizophrenia in affected families (Baron, et al., 1983; Kendler, et al., 1981a, 1984; Kety, 1983; Siever and Gunderson, 1983; Wender, et al., 1974). It seems probable that schizoid and schizotypal personality disorders result from less severe exposures to factors that cause schizophrenia (Gottesman and Shields, 1982). Finally, many schizophrenics are schizoid or schizotypal before they become psychotic (Lehmann and Cancro, 1985; Slater and Roth, 1969). If their psychoses remit, they are once again clinically schizoid or schizotypal.

The abnormalities shown by schizoids and schizotypals, as well as by schizophrenics, are easy to describe in social-strategic terms: they represent increasingly severe failures to manifest dispositions needed for mutualism and reciprocal altruism. Persons with these disorders perceive themselves to be outside their social group. They lack the positive affect and sense of camaraderie other people feel in a tight-knit social group. Lacking in trust, and without a sense of camaraderie, they tend to withdraw from everyone except their immediate family. Other social strategies, which may remain intact, continue in evidence with the immediate family. To one degree or another schizoid, schizotypal, or schizophrenic patients fail to heed reality, as their group defines it. Rather than being consensual, their thoughts are highly subjective and difficult to communicate. They may be indifferent to making themselves understood.

Jaspers (1963) thought that schizoid social withdrawal led to autistic thinking. His position is supported by recent studies that implicate social withdrawal as the primary deficit in schizotypal disorders (see Siever and Klar, 1986). Continuous social feedback may be required to suppress what we recognize as autistic thinking. Also, Cutting and Murphy (1988) showed that some of the abnormalities apparent in schizophrenic thinking result from marked deficiencies in everyday social knowledge.

Consistent with the attenuation of group-related feelings, schizoids, schizotypals, and schizophrenics tend to migrate away from their social groups (see, for example, Dunham, 1976), a move made with difficulty by more normal persons. Some of these persons become hermits or transients, in this way avoiding social groups altogether. Schizoid mobility may partly account for the high incidence of schizophrenia among immigrants (Eitinger, 1960), in rural areas (Dohrenwend and Dohrenwend, 1974), and in urban slums (Farris and Dunham, 1939; Dohrenwend and Dohrenwend, 1974; Goodman, et al., 1983).

I noted above that schizoid and schizotypal disorders are genetically inherited alongside schizophrenia in affected families. Therefore, biological factors must be acting, in concert with environmental factors, to cause social withdrawal and autistic thinking. Perceptual, cognitive, or affective abnormalities resulting from nervous dysfunction may cause miscarriage of strategies related to social groups. To mention one possibility: schizophrenics, and many schizoid and schizotypal patients as well, have difficulty interpreting and producing nonverbal social cues, especially those dependent on facial expression and eye contact (see Anstadt and Krause, 1989; Grumet, 1983; Krause, et al., 1989; Pilowsky and Bassett, 1980). By impairing affective relationships within the social group, communicational deficits might lead to widespread changes in group-related behaviors. A similar hypothesis has been proposed with regard to autistic children (see Ricks and Wing, 1975; Tinbergen and Tinbergen, 1972; cf. Tantam, 1988a, 1988b on Asperger's Syndrome). Brothers (1989) notes the role of the amygdala in interpreting social gestures. In nonhuman primates, amygdaloid and related orbito-frontal lesions sometimes produce decrements in affiliative behavior that resemble, superficially, schizoid withdrawal in humans (Butter, et al., 1970; Jacobson, 1986; Kling, 1972, 1986; Kling and Steklis, 1976; Raleigh and Steklis, 1981; Raleigh, et al., 1979). Operated-upon animals show communicational deficits, and, in certain environments, they avoid social contacts. I have already noted that certain chronic psychotics appear to have abnormalities of prefrontal regions.

Regardless of their biologic causes, schizoid and schizotypal disorders are likely to be worsened by social conditions that loosen the hold of the group on its constituent members. When group boundaries or consensual reality are blurred, individuals predisposed to feel apart from the group or to ignore consensual reality may manifest these dispositions to a greater degree. Epidemiologic evidence regarding schizophrenia is consistent with this hypothesis. The incidence of schizophrenia has apparently increased in recently Westernized regions of the third world (see, for example, Dunham, 1976; Torrey, 1979). In light of the relation between schizophrenia and schizoid and schizotypal personalities, the latter may also have increased with rapid cultural change. Westernization and urbanization break down community bonds and weaken consensual world views found in traditional cultures. Along the same lines, schizophrenics in traditional cultures, and presumably schizoids and schizotypals as well, have a better prognosis than those who live in industrial cultures (McGlashan, 1986; Sartorius, et al., 1978; Strauss and Carpenter, 1981; Verghese, et al., 1989; Warner, 1983; Waxler, 1979). More clearcut group boundaries, consensual world views, and group expectations may produce the difference.

Family studies show that lack of clarity in communications seems to be characteristic of "schizophrenic" families (Doane, et al., 1981; McGlashan, 1986; Wynne, et al., 1979). Communicational deviance might result from autistic thinking and, by impairing opportunities for consensual modeling, contribute to it as well. Numerous studies have shown that psychotherapy which increases the salience of consensual reality is helpful to schizophrenics, schizoids, and schizotypals (see, for example, Gunderson, 1979; McGlashan, 1986; Mosher and Gunderson, 1979). Psychotherapy which increases introspection, on the other hand, is unlikely to help and may even harm these patients.

Schizoids and schizotypals are oftentimes creative. For example, Hartmann (1984; Hartmann, et al., 1981) studied persons who experience frequent nightmares. Many of them were schizoid or schizotypal and also very creative. Hartmann argued that these subjects have what he called "weak boundaries." Weak boundaries make them creative but also render them vulnerable to schizophrenic psychosis. In Hartmann's view, artistic or creative pursuits protect against mental illness, so that schizotypes lacking in talent will more likely deteriorate than those with unusual gifts. Studies of schizophrenics and their close relatives are consistent with Hartmann's view. Schizophrenics themselves tend to be uncreative and lacking in specialized talents (see Rabin, et al., 1979). However, their non-psychotic relatives are frequently quite creative and are often found to be gifted (see Anthony, 1968; Heston and Denny, 1969; Karlsson, 1966; Kauffman, et al., 1979; cf. Schuldberg, et al., 1988).

The social strategic viewpoint explains the connection between schizotypal thinking and creativity. Schizotypal thinking is remarkable for its freedom from the consensual norm. Schizotypal persons are relatively unconstrained by their group's world view. If they are mildly schizotypal—that is, if they make a sufficiently good connection with the consensual world to make themselves understood— they may voice ideas new to those around them, creative ideas, in other words. Park (1928) expressed a similar notion: the so-called marginal man. The marginal man, as Park defined him, subscribes only partly to any particular culture. He may live at the boundary of two or more groups and be partly acculturated to both. Park argued that marginal men are especially likely to play creative roles leading to cultural change.

Paranoia

Schizoid or schizotypal persons are frequently paranoid (Siever and Klar, 1986). I noted above that fearfulness is part of the schizoid pattern. Paranoid personalities are, of course, also fearful, but they tend to be less isolative and to show less autistic thinking (Siever and Klar, 1986). If they become psychotic, they tend to develop delusions with a more paranoid than schizophreniform content (see Kendler and Hays, 1981; Kendler, et al., 1981b, 1985; Magaro, 1981; cf. Watt, 1985a, 1985b). Actually, schizotypal and paranoid personalities are frequently hard to distinguish (Kass, et al., 1985).

It is easy to see why schizoids are prone to paranoid feelings. Mutualism and reciprocal altruism depend on a sense of camaraderie. People within a social group feel that they are friends, and they trust each other. Schizoids and schizotypes lack a sense of camaraderie and the trust that goes with it.

In considering paranoia, it is important to keep in mind that human beings are, in fact, very dangerous animals, both in a group and individually. A prudent extraterrestrial, unless he came from a planet with even lower standards than ours, would no doubt be reluctant to wander unprotected in most human societies. Even if he disguised himself to appear as a human being, he would still be in some danger. In the following sections I will note that conflicts occur between human beings, and that in most cultures some of these may cause violence. It may be that human beings are able to live with each other only because realistic fears are outweighed by positive feelings. These positive feelings promote adherence to strategies like those discussed in this chapter, without which homo sapiens would be a dispersed territorial species, not a gregarious one. The schizoid individual, though, has less intense positive feeling toward those in his social group, and so is left with fear that has not been sufficiently neutralized. Tinbergen and Tinbergen (1972) offered a similar notion regarding autistic children.

Group motifs are evident in certain paranoid fears. For example, paranoids often feel endangered, not just by individuals, but by groups of people they believe have conspired against them. Conservative paranoids may fear the Communist Party. Protestant paranoids may fear the Catholic Church.

Certain social conditions promote paranoid feelings. These conditions interfere with the sense of camaraderie with the social group. For example, like schizophrenia, paranoid psychoses tend to be common in immigrants (Eitinger, 1960; Kendler, 1982). Paranoid psychoses are also common in those transiently living outside their native society (see, for example, Allodi, 1982). In these cases, linguistic barriers seem to be important. Oral communication is an obvious means to maintain a sense of belonging. Paranoid ideas oftentimes occur in the elderly deaf, if they lose the ability to follow conversations (see Christenson and Blazer, 1984; Herbert and Jacobson, 1967; Kay and Roth, 1961; cf. Watt, 1985a). Galanter (1983) has noted that paranoid feelings are common among those who have recently left cohesive religious groups.

Male paranoids frequently fear threats to their masculinity or sexual assaults by other men (see Rudden, et al., 1983). For example, Schreber, whose biography Freud (1911) analyzed, believed that God was making him a woman, in order to procreate with him. Niederland (1959a, 1959b) more recently uncovered additional data on Schreber's life. Based on Schreber's biography, Freud hypothesized that paranoids repress homosexual wishes. Later psychoanalysts applied Freud's hypothesis to female paranoids too (see, for example, Brenner, 1939; Thomas, 1932). There is less evidence, though, that female paranoids do have fears related to gender identity and homosexual themes (Rudden, et al., 1983).

In humans and other primates, effeminate sexual postures signify male submission (see Roth, 1971; Clutton-Brock and Harvey, 1976; Hinde and Stevenson-Hinde, 1976; Kummer, 1979; cf. Freud, 1923). For example, nonhuman primate males excluded from male groups habitually adopt a lordotic, "receptive" posture, as a way of deflecting aggression. Insofar as human males "speak" the same primitive body language as other primate males, men who feel demeaned by their social group may feel pressured to play a "receptive" role in relation to other men. This could be the source of gender-identity fears of male paranoid patients. To see how group extrusion and sexual role are linked, readers are referred to Fox (1980), who described American Indian rites pertaining to the berdache. The berdache was a male who failed his test of manhood. He was allowed to stay with the tribe only if, thereafter, he dressed and lived like a woman. Social roles like the berdache are found in other cultures (see, for example, Shepherd, 1978; Wikan, 1977, 1978).

Other manifestations of paranoid concern with social group status are expressed in more modern idioms and are thus more readily understood. Paranoids often complain that they have been somehow slighted, that others have failed to recognize their true worth and qualities (American Psychiatric Association, 1987). They account for what they see as their persecution by citing ideas of grandeur. They claim to be playing a crucial role in the politics or history of their social group, against much opposition. In this way they resolve the apparent contradiction between being an ordinary member of a social group, which is what they appear to be, and the victim of a plot mounted by other group members. Authoritarian types (see Adorno, et al., 1950; cf. Tajfel, 1979) combine paranoid thinking with overconcern about social rank. They are notable for their tendency to see every problem in in-group, out-group terms.

It is of incidental interest that paranoid anxiety, or the fear that results from doubting that members of one's social group have benign intentions, can readily be conveyed through the medium of motion pictures. A number of frightening movies work their emotional effects by allowing members of the audience, who are presumably normal, a glimpse of what it feels like to have paranoid delusions. These movies rely on the latent capacity to experience group-related fears in the same way other movies rely on the latent capacity to experience fears of heights or snakes, in order to scare the audience. One of the most effective of this genre of frightening film is the most recent version of the science fiction classic, *The Invasion of the Body Snatchers*. The protagonist in this film moves through a world of persons who appear to be friendly members of his social group, but who in fact belong to a group with hostile intentions toward him. Although they appear familiar, they are aliens to the protagonist; they come from the unknown territory beyond the familiar social group, from outer space itself!

Within-Group Conflict

Life in the mutualistic group is not entirely harmonious. In the previous chapter, I noted that conflicts occur between parents and children over parental aid. There are also within-group conflicts due to competition for limited resources which are reproductively useful. Before describing these conflicts, though, I note some important ideas concerning conflict in general.

An individual engaged in a conflict will adhere to a strategy that guides conflict behavior. If nothing else, he or she will wind up adhering to one or another strategy for varying lengths of time. For example, an individual may threaten and bluff, backing down only if an opponent escalates to the point where injury might occur. An individual may have different levels of risk he or she would incur before backing down. Or the individual may escalate himself, either spontaneously, or in measured response to escalation by others. He or she may escalate indefinitely, or to some preset limit.

A number of authors have studied animal conflict strategies from a theoretical view (see, for example, Bishop, et al., 1978; Hammerstein, 1981; Maynard Smith, 1974, 1976a, 1982b; Maynard Smith and Parker, 1976; Maynard Smith and Price, 1973; Parker, 1974, 1982). Game theory, a branch of mathematics initially developed for economic analysis, has proven especially useful when applied to animal conflicts (for overviews of game theory, see Davis, 1983; Owen, 1982; Shubik, 1982). In general, the best strategic option varies from conflict to conflict, depending upon the value of resources at stake and what others are likely to do. Perceived relative power is especially important. In commonsense terms, individuals who (rightly) perceive that they are more powerful than their potential opponents are able to choose strategies that ensure them a maximal gain. They might, for instance, escalate conflicts beyond the point their opponents can tolerate. Individuals who (rightly) perceive that they are less powerful than their potential opponents are able to choose strategies that ensure them a minimal loss. If nothing else, they can avoid injuries sustained in battles they were destined to lose. Individuals who cannot correctly perceive their relative power are unable to make strategic choices that optimize either their gains or losses.

Conflicts are so frequent, and determine access to such crucial resources, that even small advantages in choosing conflict strategies will have major effects on inclusive fitness.

Relative power may be evident. One party to a conflict, for instance, may be obviously stronger than others. If relative power isn't evident, members of many species will engage in ritual combat or other displays of power (for examples, see Eibl-Eibesfeldt, 1970). Ritual combat and displays allow potential combatants to exchange information needed to optimize outcome without the risk of injury attendant on all-out fighting. All-out fighting will ensue only if ritual combat and displays convince both combatants to further escalate conflict.

Parker (1974) coined the term Resource Holding Power (RHP) to signify estimates of relative power with respect to opponents. The term correctly implies that the major source of conflicts for which power is needed are resource disputes. That is, two or more individuals seek a limited quantity of useful resources.

As I noted in chapter 3, human conflicts are most often fought out in the social arena, not in physical combat. Consequently, human RHP is less determined by physical size and strength than by social relationships. Authority, prestige, wealth, birthright, and family ties determine RHP in human communities. Charisma and intelligence are more important to human power than physical prowess.

I noted too that determinants of human RHP are also the major determinants of self-esteem. Social skills, charisma, intelligence, and position increase self-esteem as well as RHP. Both self-esteem and RHP increase with successes in the social realm. Failures lower RHP and self-esteem together. Self-esteem may be the subjective counterpart to RHP. Writing on a related theme, cognitive therapists have emphasized the importance of what people believe about themselves, and in particular, what they believe about their own competencies (see, for example, Abramson, et al., 1978; Bandura, 1977; Bandura, et al., 1977; Beck, 1972, 1976; Beck, et al., 1974; Costello, 1978; Ellis, 1962; Ellis and Grieger, 1977; Rizley, 1978; Seligman, 1975; Weintraub, et al., 1974)). In chapter 3, I noted that what Bandura (1977) called "self-efficacy" is related to RHP and affects aid-seeking behaviors. Human RHP depends upon social and other skills of the most varied kind. These skills determine self-efficacy. On the other hand, humans are too thoroughly social to consider that their feelings of self-efficacy could be divorced from power applied in the social arena. This power determines perceived RHP. Thus, RHP, self-efficacy and self-esteem are interrelated constructs. RHP, self-efficacy, or self-esteem must exert control over strategic decisions.

Male Reproductive Strategies

In any species, members of the sex capable of producing the greatest number of offspring compete with each other for the opportunity to mate (Clutton-Brock and Harvey, 1976; Trivers, 1972). Given a limited number of the less prolific sex, a member of the potentially more prolific sex can realize his or her reproductive potential only by obtaining more than his or her share of mates. The intensity of competition depends on the difference in reproductive capacities of the two sexes (see, for example, Wiley, 1973; LeBoeuf, 1974). Because the human male can sire many more children than any woman can bear, competition between men should be a substantive factor in human social relations.

Men are generally eager to have sexual intercourse. Contraceptive methods have loosened the link between sex and reproduction, so men cannot really be said to adhere any longer to a reproductive strategy by seeking sexual intercourse. However, before the invention of contraceptive methods, seeking sexual intercourse was an effective means to use reproductive capacity of the opposite sex. Consistent with their desire for intercourse per se, men are most often attentive to sexual opportunities of the most casual kind. In this respect they differ from the average woman (see Mellen, 1981; Symons, 1979, for reviews). Symons (1979) observed that while men are generally aroused by cues suggesting a woman is available, women are more often aroused by cues suggesting a loving relationship (see also Steinman, et al., 1981). Male homosexuals, who can express the pattern of sexual activity preferred by males without having to compromise with female sexual preferences, are frequently promiscuous. Promiscuous homosexual men may have hundreds of partners by the time they are middle aged (Symons, 1979). Lesbians, by contrast, tend to form sexually faithful long-term relationships (see also, Bell and Weinberg, 1978; Saghir and Robins, 1973; Tollison and Adams, 1979).

In most societies, men compete with each other to attain power or status, which is linked to sexual access. In many societies, men with the greatest social rank enjoy multiple wives, concubines, or mistresses (see Chagnon, 1974, 1979a, 1980; Chagnon, et al., 1979; Cohen, 1961; Irons, 1979, 1980, 1983; Malinowski, 1961; Murdock, 1967). Men with the least social rank may fail to marry at all. In hunter-gatherer groups like those in which humans evolved, male social success and reproductive success are very highly correlated. Small groups of powerful men may literally determine the genetic composition of later generations. In modern western societies, middle and upper class men and their wives may limit their family size, but even in these societies, higher social class apparently protects men against the failure to reproduce (see Essock-Vitale, 1983; Kunz, et al., 1973; Tiger, 1979). In any event, limitations on family size may be understandable in ecological terms. When resources are predictable, reproductive fitness may ultimately be maximized by having fewer children who are very intensively reared (cf. Davis and Blake, 1956; Gadgil and Bossert, 1970; Lack, 1954, 1966, 1968; MacArthur and Wilson, 1967; Pianka, 1970; Reynolds and Tanner, 1983; Stearns, 1977, 1982). Low fertility rates with intensive parental investments in children were very likely typical of prehistoric societies, as they are of modern hunter-gatherer tribes (Draper and Harpending, 1988; Short, 1976).

Males compete with each other in an arena—economic or political—defined by social mores. In this way societies harness the motive force provided by male desire. A similar process also occurs for women (see below). Although sexual tributaries to various social ambitions most often go unacknowledged, the process noted here differs from "sublimation" in the Freudian sense (see Brenner, 1974; Fenichel, 1945; Freud, 1905). Sublimation entails giving up sexual aims.

Male competition occasionally spills out of the socially sanctioned arena and leads to violence. In some primitive societies, a significant number of men may die from murder and warfare (see, for example, Symons, 1979; Chagnon, 1977; Chagnon and Bugos, 1979). Primitive murder and warfare are frequently over women. Primitive women, by contrast, less frequently perpetrate or fall victim to violence (Burbank, 1987). In modern societies, almost all violent criminals are men dissatisfied with what they can achieve by conventional means. By contrast, violent female criminals tend to be mentally ill (Wilson and Herrnstein, 1985). In effect, modern societies arm themselves against dissatisfied males.

In most societies, selective pressures dictate that women mate with men who are able and willing to help care for children (see below). In these societies, female inclusive fitness is diminished by casual mating, or by mating with men who will not reliably aid their children (cf. Orians, 1969; Symons, 1979; Trivers, 1972). Because women in these societies more readily mate with men who have resources needed for rearing children, male competition may be played out in a struggle for resource control. Resource control can be achieved politically or by acquiring wealth. Irons (1979, 1980) found that birth rates and childhood mortality rates varied with wealth in the cultures he studied. Wealthier parents apparently used their resources to effectively aid their children. Infant and child mortality and family poverty are strongly associated even in Western countries (S. Klein, 1980).

Standards of beauty, jealousy, and many other aspects of male sexual life in particular societies are wholly or partially explicable with inclusive fitness models (see, for example, Buss, 1987, 1989; Daly and Wilson, 1987; Symons, 1979; R. Thornhill and Thornhill, 1983, 1987; Townsend, 1989). These topics, however, are beyond the scope of this study.

Female Reproductive Strategies

In any species, members of the less prolific sex should readily fulfill their reproductive capacity. Members of the opposite sex compete to help them do so! Therefore, members of the less prolific sex will devote their efforts not so much to producing more, but to ensuring that the offspring they do have reach reproductive maturity and are capable of mating (cf. Orians, 1969; Symons, 1979; Trivers, 1972). Offspring who perish or who are incapable of mating use up limited reproductive capacity but do not increase parental fitness (see chapter 2). In homo sapiens, females are the less prolific sex. And, consistent with their limited reproductive capacity, women most often play the major role in seeing that children survive. As noted in the previous chapter, mothers are most often the primary attachment figures for their own children.

Though they often end up raising children alone, women in most societies try to guarantee they will have some masculine help. They do so by selectively mating with men who are able and willing to provide paternal aid (see Buss, 1987, 1989; Townsend, 1989). By selecting potential fathers who control useful resources, and who show a propensity to devote those resources to children, women can insure that their future children enjoy the benefits of paternal aid. These benefits can be substantial; in many societies, available paternal aid, in addition to maternal care, determines whether a child lives and is able to later mate. It is important to note again that male resource control is not a simple matter. Males control resources by virtue of social position, long-standing social contracts, including property rights, and political alliances with other adults in the social group. They do not control resources by solitary exercise of physical strength, nor in opposition to all potential competitors, who would simply band against them.

Insofar as they depend on male parental aid in order to raise their children, women must provide their mates with evidence of paternity. Men willing to devote resources to children without evidence that they are the fathers would suffer decreased fitness, in comparison with men who expect some proof of paternity. In male-dominated societies, women typically offer men evidence for their paternity by disavowing sexual interests in general, and certainly sexual interests in other men, or by submitting to claustration and other restrictive rules (see below).

In many societies females are prevented from controlling any resources at all so that they are wholly dependent on male parental aid, and resources are concentrated so that only a few males control sufficient resources to effectively aid their children. In order to guarantee that their future children survive, women in such societies must compete with each other for mates who control resources. Hypergamy, the tendency for especially attractive women to marry up in social class, and polygynous marriage rules that allow powerful men more than one wife, have been widely observed in stratified societies dominated by men (see, for example, Buss, 1987, 1989; Dickemann, 1979; N.W. Thornhill and Thornhill, 1987).

Inclusive fitness arguments predict that human female sexual competition will remain nonviolent, compared to competition occurring between men (Trivers, 1972). This is not to say that female competition is not pervasive and energetic, just that the inclusive fitness stakes are such that it rarely pays individuals to risk serious injury in a single encounter (cf. Hrdy, 1981). I have already noted disparities in male and female violence consistent with this prediction (see Burbank, 1987). Sex-related differences in size and aggressiveness support the same conclusion (see below).

In most male-dominated societies, men accrue resources as they mature. Consequently, in selecting mates able to care for their children, women in these societies appear to find attractive men somewhat older than they are. By contrast, men of any age are sexually attracted most strongly by young women, the latter being at or near their reproductive prime (see, for example, Buss, 1987, 1989; Mead, 1967; Symons, 1979; Townsend, 1989; Williams, 1975).

In some societies, coalitions of female kin are sufficiently productive to forgo male assistance in rearing children (Irons, 1979, 1983; Leacock, 1978, 1980; cf. Whyte, 1978). As a consequence, women in these societies are less restricted sexually than women in societies dominated by men. Also, men in these societies seek competent, powerful women able to offer them aid. Societies like these may have been more common before intergroup warfare, which promotes male dominance, became a chronic condition (see above, also Leacock, 1978, 1980; cf. Schmookler, 1984; Tiger, 1984). Similar social structures are found among nonhuman primates (see, for example, Hrdy, 1981; Silk and Boyd, 1983). Certain western societies appear to be in the process of turning back the clock. Women may soon control resources needed for raising children without paternal aid. If this occurs, new sexual mores and altered mating preferences can be expected to follow.

Sexual and reproductive strategies contingent on environmental factors have been described in many animal species (Draper and Harpending, 1988; R. Thornhill and Thornhill, 1983, 1987). Draper and Harpending (1982, 1988; see also Blain and Barkow, 1988) suggest that the contingent cue determining human female reproductive strategy is the presence or absence of the father in the female child's environment during a critical period. Women raised with paternal assistance pursue reproductive strategies aimed at obtaining male aid. Women raised without paternal assistance pursue reproductive strategies that do not depend on male aid. Draper and Harpending's thesis has obvious implications for the effects of divorce on later social arrangements (see chapter 5).

In many societies, maternal uncles contribute to rearing their nieces and nephews. This may occur when the certainty of paternity is low, so that husbands cannot be sure if their wives' children are their own (Kurland, 1979). By helping to rear children of uterine sisters, men direct their aid toward recipients who are certainly their genetic kin. In these societies too, women can choose husbands without concern for ability to provide paternal aid, in spite of the fact that they themselves may not control resources.

Patterns of arousal, infidelity, jealousy, and other aspects of female sexual life are also intelligible in terms of inclusive fitness (see, for example, Symons, 1979). Arousal is discussed below. Suffice it to say here that women dependent on male paternal assistance should generally be slower to become sexually aroused than males, should be sexually more faithful to their mates than men, and should be jealous of their mates' affections. Women not dependent on male paternal assistance might be more readily aroused, less faithful, and less concerned with their mates' affections than women dependent on men.

Both male and female reproductive strategies are evolutionarily stable. Men who fail to compete with other men to please women— by controlling resources or by other means—will have less use of female reproductive potential. Women dependent on paternal assistance who take as their mates competitively unsuccessful men will give birth to children who will later be disadvantaged. Being at least contingently universal and evolutionarily stable, male and female reproductive strategies are innately probable in the sense described in chapter 2.

Innate Dispositions
Promoting Reproductive Strategies

Obviously, heterosexual preferences promote adherence to both male and female reproductive strategies. Not surprisingly, these preferences depend in part on innate events. For example, animal studies have shown that parts of the nervous system differentiate early in life along male or female lines. Among other factors, fetal gonadal hormones affect the developing brain. Nervous system commitment apparently helps determine later sexual preference (for reviews of nervous system commitment, see Ehrhardt and Meyer-Bahlburg, 1981; Goy and McEwan, 1980; Gray and Drewett, 1977; Herbert, 1976; MacLusky and Naftolin, 1981; Resko, 1975; Schumacher and Balthazart, 1985; Schumacher, et al., 1987).

The discovery that the nervous system differentiates early into male or female lines has increased interest in the biological basis of homosexual object choice (see, for example, Dorner, 1976, 1980). Environmental theories of homosexual object choice have generally not been supported by empirical studies (see, for example, Bell, et al., 1981).

I noted above that men and women differ in their patterns of sexual arousal. Rapid arousal promotes adherence to the male sexual strategy: to use as much female reproductive capacity as possible. Somewhat slower arousal, contingent on loving relationships, promotes adherence to the female sexual strategy: to be selective in choice of mates, at least in conditions where paternal aid is needed. Innately controlled hormones and neurotransmitters affect sexual interest (see, for example, Charney and Heninger, 1986; Clark, et al., 1984; Gessa and Tagliomonte, 1974; Harvey, 1988; Margolis, et al., 1971; Mirin, et al., 1980; Rubin, et al., 1981; Schiavi, 1981; Schumacher, et al., 1987). Some of these are known to differ between the sexes and to be responsive to psychosocial conditions.

The male's greater reproductive advantage in becoming rapidly aroused helps to explain why most fetishists are male (see Tollison and Adams, 1979). Although some signs of female receptiveness—such as certain unclothed postures—are universal, most are culture–specific. This has no doubt been the case for hundreds of generations. In order for males to take advantage of sexual opportunities, male arousal must be readily conditioned to culture–specific contingencies. Ready conditionability leads to a risk of fetishism with objects associated with sexual satisfaction (cf. Rachman, 1968; Rachman and Hodgson, 1968).

The vast majority of voyeurs are men, too (Tollison and Adams, 1979). In many societies, and to a certain extent in our own, female nudity signifies receptiveness. Therefore, men in these societies are readily aroused by the sight of the female body, or even by seeing bodily parts—such as a foot or ankle—normally covered by garments. Arousal can become conditioned to peeping behaviors. On the other hand, consistent with their own reproductive strategy, women in these societies are less aroused by nakedness than by erotic overtures in a loving relationship (see Symons, 1979). Unlike men, for instance, modern American women evince little interest in pictorial pornography that merely shows naked bodies.

I noted above that although their sexual strategies may require that both men and women compete with others of their sex, male competition is more likely to lead to violence. Consequently, greater innate aggressiveness might promote male sexual strategies. In their well-known review, Maccoby and Jacklin (1974) did consider aggressiveness a male characteristic independent of culture. Men are larger than women, suggesting that ancestral males relied on force or the threat of force to further their reproduction (cf. Trivers, 1972), and men are more likely to both commit and fall victim to acts of lethal violence (see above). Neurotransmitters, hormones, and certain brain structures are known to play roles in determining male aggressiveness (see, for example, Eichelman, 1986). Particular attention has been paid to hormone levels, which differ between the sexes. As well as enhancing sexual drive, high androgen levels may predispose to aggressiveness (see Eichelman, 1986; Maccoby and Jacklin, 1974; Olweus, et al., 1988; Rubin, et al., 1981; Schumacher, et al., 1987). In rhesus monkeys, androgen hormone levels affect male dominance rankings (Rose, Gordon, and Bernstein, 1971, 1972; Rose, Holaday, and Bernstein, 1971).

However, even before puberty, both human and nonhuman primate infants show sex-related differences in their aggressive play (see, for example, Lawick-Goodall, 1971; Kummer, 1968). Before puberty, gonadal hormone levels are normally low in both sexes. Evidence suggests that early nervous system commitment may affect later aggressiveness, as it does sexual preference (see, for example, Conner, et al., 1969; Ehrhardt and Meyer-Bahlburg, 1981; Meyer-Bahlburg, et al., 1988; Yalom, et al., 1973).

Generalized Sexual Inhibitions

Most clinicians agree that generalized sexual inhibitions can produce psychological problems. Psychological problems related to these inhibitions may occur less frequently now than two or three decades ago, but they are still often encountered in everyday clinical practice. Ethnographers have shown that generalized sexual inhibitions are not really universal; they occur in societies when parents or other authorities discourage young children from expressing sexual interest (see, for example, Firth, 1957; Fortes, 1949; Malinowski, 1927,

1932; Mead, 1950). But why do some parents or other authority figures discourage developing sexual interest in the most general sense? Why should adults inhibit feelings that lead their offspring to procreate? I will address this question in inclusive fitness terms. Specific sexual prohibitions are discussed in the following section.

First, a woman who has a child who cannot be cared for decreases not only her own, but also her parents' fitness. If mothers need spousal assistance, the only way for women to see that their children are cared for is to bear children in "marriage," however that is defined in their particular culture. Parents in these societies should not want their daughters to have "premarital" pregnancies.

In many societies, parents trade virginal daughters for other women or property (see, for example, Daly and Wilson, 1979). This makes it doubly important that unmarried daughters be chaste, to prevent them from giving away what can be traded for profit. According to Levi-Strauss (1969), the male urge to trade daughters and other female kin for unrelated women plays a pivotal role in forming human society (see also, Chagnon, 1979b; Fox, 1979).

Second, a sexually unfaithful woman may decrease her husband's fitness. If she becomes pregnant by another man, she denies her spouse access to her reproductive potential. If her spouse does not know that he has become a cuckold, he may help raise a child who carries another man's genes.

Therefore, if fathers contribute substantially to child-rearing, both "husbands" and parents with daughters benefit by curbing female sexual interest. And in fact, in societies characterized by large paternal investments in children—and relative female dependence— parents train young women to suppress their sexual urges. With expectations and sanctions, husbands in these societies reinforce this training. Parents and husbands use ethical mores to effectively increase their fitness (see chapter 2). Parents can rest assured that their pure and virginal daughters will save their reproductive potential for their legitimate mates, who will help care for their children. Husbands can rest assured that their chaste wives will be faithful. In these societies, women who are lustful may be considered unmarriageable.

It is worth noting that in particular cultures, more extreme steps might be taken to curb female sexual life. Though these may be aberrations, they illustrate the importance of female sexuality to parents and future husbands. For example, parents in some societies clitoridectomize daughters (see, for example, Hathout, 1963; Mustafa, 1966). Because clitoridectomy decreases pleasure in later sexual acts, clitoridectomized women are thought to be more chaste (Trimingham, 1949). Clitoral cauterization and even clitoridectomy were occasionally carried out by nineteenth century doctors trying to "cure" masturbation (Bullough and Bullough, 1977).

It is somewhat less clear why men should be trained to have sexual inhibitions. Of course, in spite of the "double standard" typical of societies in which men make the decisions, men may be caught inadvertently in a moral net intended mainly for women. It may not be possible to teach one sex that lust is something degraded without giving a similar message to the opposite sex. This is especially true since sons are trained to consider lustful women degraded, and consequently unmarriageable, as a means of defense against cuckoldry. Also, in most societies, advantageous marriages are based on factors unrelated to mere sexual interest (see Symons, 1979). Freedom of sexual interest might lead young men to make otherwise foolish marital choices, reducing their parents' fitness. Parents should therefore benefit by restricting their sons' freedom to express sexual interest, just as they do with their daughters. If nothing else, inhibiting sons' sexuality to conform with restrictive mores might decrease the chance of conflict with other men in the group (see above).

When women control resources needed for raising children, neither parents nor husbands may have compelling reasons to limit female sexual life, or to propagate sexual ideologies. In fact, societies in which women wield productive power are generally less prudish with regard to sexual matters (see, for example, Irons, 1979, 1983; Leacock, 1978, 1980; Whyte, 1978). Though specific matings may be proscribed, sexuality in general is neither shamed nor inhibited. In western countries, the sexual revolution occurred about the same time as women obtained greater freedom to make their way in the world.

More than any other psychiatric disorder, hysteria has been thought to be due to sexual urges subject to inhibitions. For example, Freud (1905) thought that the young woman he called Dora was sexually attracted to a male friend of the family. Dora's hysterical symptoms were said to express her desire in symbolic form. For classical psychoanalysts, Dora has served as a model of how sexual urges might produce conversion and other hysterical symptoms.

More recently, however, studies of patients with hysterical features have emphasized their dependency and what might be called their attachment needs. Marmor (1954), for example, described "oral hysterics," whose hysterical symptomatology seemed to him to be due to passive dependency and early oral drives. In recent years, investigators have described so-called hysteroid dysphorics, who resemble hysterical personalities, are dependent and clinging, and respond to losses with severe depression (Klein, 1975; Stone, 1980). Depression has been shown to be common in hysterical patients (see, for example, Ziegler, et al., 1960; Zoccolillo and Cloninger, 1986). Studies of well-known hysterics described by Charcot clearly indicate that they suffered severe early losses and other traumatic experiences now thought to affect later attachment needs (see Drinka, 1984).

Draper and Harpending (1988) argued that, by exaggerating their neediness to men, self-dramatizing hysterical women pursue an exploitative variant of the normal female reproductive strategy, which is, at least in most societies, to seek male assistance needed for rearing children. Draper and Harpending's argument and clinical experience linking hysteria to dependency might be reconciled if hysterical women are using a female reproductive strategy to meet their attachment needs. However, Draper and Harpending expressly state that their argument applies to Briquet's Hysteria, in which somatic complaints are the means of seeking attention (see Goodwin and Guze, 1984). I noted in chapter 3 that children may feign illness and incapacity in order to increase rates of parental aid. If somatization in Briquet's Hysteria is analogous to behaviors in early attachment relationships in that they both serve to gain assistance, it is hard to see what is specifically sexual about Briquet's Hysteria, except the fact that it is most often found in women. But somatization and hysterical traits also occur in men (Luisada, et al., 1974), and in any event, sex differences in diagnosis of hysteria may be a reflection of cultural opportunities to meet attachment needs in other ways, rather than the result of differences in reproductive strategies. Data indicating that patriarchal cultures produce women with hysterical features (Chodoff, 1982; Weller, 1988) are consistent with the notion that hysteria is a disease resulting in large part from power-lessness. Many women with Briquet's syndrome are sexually pro-miscuous, but promiscuity is also frequently seen in borderline personality, which I have argued is due to attachment events (see chapter 3).

Draper and Harpending's argument that Briquet's Hysteria is an alternate reproductive strategy rests in part on evidence that it is related to male antisocial personality disorder (see, for example, Goodwin and Guze, 1984), which they also conceive of as a repro-ductive strategy. However, Warner (1978) argued that antisocial and hysterical personalities have similar psychodynamics that are more closely related to issues of neediness and self-worth than to purely sexual issues, and that are expressed in different forms by men and women (see also Vaillant, 1975).

In any event, any patient with hysterical features will be sexually provocative, self-dramatizing, or dependent, and will show somati-zation to some degree or another. The combination of elements, together with personal histories, may allow for a formulation in each individual case. The syndrome may appear to be a rather pure expression of attachment needs, an expression of attachment needs in the form of a reproductive strategy, or a reproductive strategy as Draper and Hapending argue.

Incest and the Oedipal Complex

Children born to closely related parents are more likely to have severe genetic defects than children born to unrelated parents (see, for example, Adams and Neel, 1967; Carter, 1967; Morton, 1958; Schull, 1958; Seemanova, 1971; Yamaguchi, et al., 1970; cf. Thomp-son, 1982). Consequently, insofar as they choose mates to maximize inclusive fitness, persons should prefer mates who are not close genetic kin. Outbreeding preferences have been observed in non-human primates (see, for example, Itoigawa, et al., 1981; Lawick-Goodall, 1971; Sade, 1968) and other animal species (see, for exam-ple, Agren, 1984; Bateson, 1978, 1982; Dewsbury, 1982; Hill, 1974; Hoogland, 1982).

There are conditions, though, in which individuals are likely to have sexual intercourse with close kin. For example, innate discriminant cues which might prevent inbreeding in the environment of adaptation may be attenuated by particular cultures, and especially by their child-rearing methods. The famous debate between Freud (1913, 1917) and Westermarck (1921, 1926, 1934a, 1934b) hinged on whether innate cues, similar to those responsible for preventing excessive inbreeding in animal species (see above), prevent sibling incest in human beings. It now appears that they do, but that they are lacking in cultures that prevent intimate physical contact between young children (see, for example, Fox, 1980; Shepher, 1983; Spiro, 1958; Talmon, 1964; Wolf, 1966, 1968, 1970; cf. Myers, 1982). The environment of adaptation is the type of social milieu in which behavior evolved.

If the environment is such that closely related genetic kin may attempt to have intercourse, their relatives should prevent it (Fox, 1980). This is because individuals can increase their inclusive fitness by keeping genetic kin from disadvantageous matings. The most efficient way to block sexual activity between close kin who are not already averse to it is to promote mores that prohibit their sexual union. Empirical studies show that strong sexual mores can in fact suppress the activities which they aim to prevent (see, for example, Herold and Goodwin, 1981; Kinsey, et al., 1948, 1953; Tavris and Sadd, 1975).

At the beginning of chapter 3 I noted issues concerning the correlation between nominal and genetic kinship. The same issues pertain to whether exogamy rules, which prohibit marriage within nominal kin groups, serve to prevent excessive genetic inbreeding. All exogamy systems do prevent matings between the closest genetic kin (see, for example, N.W. Thornhill and Thornhill, 1987; van den Berghe, 1980, 1983, 1987).

In chapter 2, I argued that moral ideologies are promoted by powerful persons who stand to benefit from them. By "powerful" I mean sufficiently powerful to inculcate and enforce a particular moral rule. For instance, parents are powerful with respect to their children. An obvious implication of the argument in chapter 2 is that people are trained to be moral precisely because they might otherwise act differently. Because the temptation to sibling incest varies from one society to another, taboos against sibling incest have proven especially helpful in illustrating this point (see Fox, 1980).

Taboos against sibling incest tend to be prominent only in societies that efface innate discriminant cues preventing sibling desire.

By studying individuals, Freud discovered that moral attitudes, and especially sexual mores, coexist together with immoral impulses (Fenichel, 1945). The models developed here indicate that inculcated moralities are founded on strong temptations that provide their raison d'etre. Where temptation is lacking, morality tends to be absent.

Gender-related differences in sexual drive explain why mother-son incest is much more rare than father-daughter incest (Cavallin, 1973; Geiser, 1979; Justice and Justice, 1979; Seemanova, 1971; Weinberg, 1955) and more indicative of severe psychopathology (Sadock, 1985). First, I noted above that men tend to be drawn to rather young women, who have more reproductive potential. Where men control resources needed for rearing children, women are often attracted to somewhat older men, who have achieved some status. Consequently, fathers may be attracted to their maturing daughters, but mothers are less likely to be attracted to sons. Second, in most societies the average man will have more driven, appetitive sexual feelings than the average woman. Male sexual feelings, moreover, are likely to be more independent of interpersonal context. With rare exceptions, parent-child incest is begun by the parent. With driven sexual feelings dependent mostly on physical cues, and finding their daughters attractive, fathers are more likely than mothers to take this critical step.

According to believers in classical Freudian theory (see Fenichel, 1945), young children experience incestuous wishes toward parents and siblings of the opposite sex. These wishes lead to conflicts—both real and fantasized—with the same sex parent. According to Freudians, furthermore, unresolved incestuous wishes lead to psychopathology. Since men or women with unresolved incestuous wishes unconsciously view sexual life as an occasion for conflict, they employ pathogenic defenses to ward off instinctual drives.

Sociobiological models suggest that Freud was wrong in attributing sexual fear and guilt to early incestuous wishes. Instead, these models suggest that intrasexual conflicts and conflicts related to mores, and their attendant anxieties, are intrinsic to sexual life. Intrasexual conflicts even occur in species in which there is no equivalent to human parental care, much less an Oedipal complex. The models described in this chapter suggest that the Oedipal complex may be a kind of rehearsal, within the family environment, for exigencies of adult life. As a rule, children practice behavior patterns that achieve their functional form only when they are grown. Sexual competition is unlikely to be an exception.

Insofar as Freud's Oedipal theory has been successful at all, it has been as a masculine rather than as a feminine psychology (see, for example, Fisher and Greenberg, 1985; Kline, 1972; Rohrbaugh, 1979). In fact, if the Oedipal complex results from preparation for later competitive strategies, it should be more salient in boys than in girls. Sexual competition is more intense and more often violent for men than for women (see above). Men have more to lose, in an inclusive fitness sense, by failing in competition for desirable mates.

As I noted above, adequate conflict behavior depends on RHP, self-esteem, or self-efficacy. These are three different terms for a cognitive "representation" of self in relation to others with whom conflicts occur. Insofar as low RHP, self-esteem, or self-efficacy impairs intrasex competition, it might lead to preoccupations with apparently Oedipal themes. Consistent with this notion, Kohut (1971, 1972, 1977, 1979, 1984) and others (see Goldberg, 1978, 1980; Kohut and Wolf, 1978; Ornstein, 1978; Tolpin, 1983) observe that some neuroses characterized by salient Oedipal issues appear to be caused by defects relating to self-esteem. In these cases, Oedipal issues abate when these defects are normalized.

Actually, Kohut and his followers discuss the state of the "Self," rather than self-esteem. Hence their approach has been called "Self Psychology." However, fluctuations in the state of the Self are manifested in part by changes in self-esteem, and self-esteem is what is pertinent here. Numerous authors have criticized Kohut's conceptual scheme, and especially his notion of a reified self (see, for example, Eagle, 1984; Gedo, 1979, 1980; Greenberg and Mitchell, 1983; Slap and Levine, 1978; Stolorow, 1976; Wallerstein, 1981, 1983, 1985).

Kohut and his followers make some points relevant to this study. First, these authors note that patients change their behavior toward others—and especially, toward their therapist—coincident with changes in their self-regard. Similar changes in response to altered RHP were discussed in the previous chapter in relation to patients who are depressed or manic. I think the cases described by Kohut and others illustrate how self-regard modulates hostile behavior in those who are already angry.

Second, according to Kohut, children achieve adequate self-regard partly by displaying themselves to responsive—or in Kohut's terminology, mirroring—parents. In chapter 3, I emphasized the proximity maintenance function of childhood self-display. In light of Kohut's observations, it seems plausible that self-display also helps the child form a realistic self-regard in relation to other people. Since accurate RHP, self-esteem, or self-efficacy is important to later success in conflict-related strategies, parents maximizing their own inclusive fitness should help the child form a realistic self-image. This should be neither grandiose nor excessively modest.

Finally, when their self-esteem was low, some of the patients described by Kohut and his followers became dependent and needy. In chapter 3 I noted that decreased RHP, self-efficacy, or self-esteem consequent on failures encountered in everyday life might evoke elements of early attachment strategies.

Many patients with disorders related to attachment strategies (chapter 3) are handicapped, too, in sexual competition. Depressed younger patients, in particular, frequently see themselves as personally or sexually inadequate in comparison with others of their sex. Expecting rejection, they avoid making overtures to the opposite sex. Oedipal themes are evident in their fears and fantasies. In these cases, decreased RHP, self-esteem, or self-efficacy promoting excessively salient early attachment strategies (see chapter 3) may be disrupting conflict-related behaviors. On the other hand, manics, who seem to have high self-efficacy (chapter 3), are often too aggressive in seeking relationships with the opposite sex.

5
Pathogenic and Curative Factors

I n previous chapters I discussed specific mental disorders familiar to clinicians. Pathogenic and curative factors were mentioned only insofar as they helped identify the social strategic correlates of particular syndromes. In this chapter I will discuss these factors in a more general way. Havens (1987) observed that psychotherapists from different schools of thought elicit different types of information from their patients. The Freudian analyst, for example, elicits information on early family life, on sexual wishes, and on dreams. The objective-descriptive psychiatrist, by contrast, elicits information mainly on symptoms and signs. Each type of therapist intervenes with the patient according to the type of data base elicited, and assesses therapeutic results by changes in that data base. In this chapter, I hope to show what type of information a sociobiologically oriented psychiatrist might try to obtain and address, as well as some of the curative factors such a psychiatrist would try to keep in mind. The topics in this chapter cannot be treated in detail, but are mentioned in order to stimulate further thinking. Specific examples are taken from earlier chapters.

According to sociobiological models, human beings adhere to social strategies which, in the past, have conferred selective advantages. Innate characteristics increase the likelihood of adherence to these strategies, at least in environments like those in which humans evolved. The most salient strategies early in life have as their ultimate aim securing aid and protection. As the individual matures, strategies of this type become progressively muted. Other strategies, with competitive, reproductive and cooperative goals, or aimed at providing aid to offspring and other kin, eventually become salient in adult behavior.

Syndromes we recognize as mental disorders correspond to dysfunctions of a few of these strategies, or of their major parts. I have tried to show, for instance, that depression, agoraphobia, borderline personality, and perhaps bipolar disease occur in the setting of dysfunctions of childhood strategies aimed at obtaining aid. For various reasons elements of these strategies remain excessively salient after the time of life in which they normally wane. Oedipal conflicts, sexual inhibitions, and deviant sexual preferences correspond to dysfunctions in reproductive strategies. Schizotypal disorders and some psychotic symptoms correspond to dysfunctions in strategies leading to membership in groups.

If mental disorders correspond to dysfunctions of social strategies, then factors affecting strategies determine mental health. Factors that decrease the likelihood of adherence to normal strategies may promote mental disorder. Correcting such factors may be prophylactically useful or even therapeutic for those already ill.

Therefore, in the course of evaluating a patient, a sociobiologically oriented clinician would try to assess factors affecting strategies relevant to the illness. In evaluating a patient with depressive illness, the important factors will be those affecting social strategies aimed at obtaining aid. In evaluating a patient with notable Oedipal conflicts or narcissistic problems, the important factors will be those affecting social strategies of a competitive, sexual type. In evaluating a schizoid, the important factors will be those affecting strategies related to the group.

A "Biopsychosocial" Approach

Modern authors on psychosomatic disorders advocate what they call a "biopsychosocial" approach (see, for example, Mattsson and Kim, 1985). Using this approach, clinicians consider biologic, psychologic, and social factors contributing to disease. Care is taken not to ignore any class of determinants.

A biopsychosocial approach is also useful in considering factors affecting social strategies. By considering systematically biologic, psychologic, and social factors affecting social strategies, we can avoid overlooking major determinants of mental health or illness, insofar as these are known in light of present-day knowledge.

I have already cited numerous biologic factors affecting social behaviors. For example, in chapter 3 I noted that emotional responses—especially separation anxiety and feelings of loss—seem to control strategies aimed at obtaining parental aid. Both in childhood and later in life, the intensity of these affects seems to be determined by biologic factors that are potentially modified by pharmacologic treatment. Clinicians frequently observe shifts in social behavior, corresponding to normalization of social strategies, following treatment of abnormal moods with psychotropic medication. Chronically depressed or anxious patients treated with medications exhibit more independence and fewer care-seeking behaviors. Hostility and energy level affect competitive strategies and seem to be determined in part by biologic factors (see chapter 4). Sexual drive and object choice were described in chapter 4 in biologic terms. Bodily form and appearance are dependent on biology. By affecting self-esteem (see, for example, Robin, et al., 1988; Weisfeld and Billings, 1988), they determine competitive strategies and aid-seeking behaviors. In chapter 5 I mentioned that forebrain dopamine systems seem to affect the salience of internal stimuli and consequently influence conformity with group beliefs. Dopamine receptor blockers seem to restore conformity, in limited respects.

In general, when social strategic deviance is genetically heritable, biologic factors must play an important role. I have already cited studies showing that virtually all the disorders discussed in previous chapters, which are manifested by social strategic dysfunction, are genetically heritable, at least to some extent.

In previous chapters, I cited psychological factors affecting social strategies. An especially important psychological factor discussed in previous chapters is self-esteem, self-efficacy, or resource holding power. I have shown how these terms are more or less interrelated. Self-efficacy determines the salience of strategies aimed at obtaining aid and the manner in which competitive strategies are expressed. Self-efficacy is affected by biologic factors, as in bipolar affective disease, and by social experience.

I noted in chapter 3 that efforts to change self-efficacy through cognitive interventions may decrease vulnerability to depression. They lead to behavioral changes consistent with decreased salience of childlike aid-seeking strategies. Interpersonal therapists also try to modify self-efficacy. They do so by calling attention to interpersonal tactics determined by low self-efficacy or to prior events affecting self-regard (see Klerman, et al., 1984). Recent trends in psychoanalysis, too, have focused greater attention on the vicissitudes of self-esteem (see chapter 4).

As I noted in chapter 4 Badcock (1986) has argued that identification, in the psychoanalytic sense, is the major proximate mechanism evolved to promote altruistic behavior in human beings. Other persons, in other words, are sufficiently incorporated into the altruist's self-representation that their needs are experienced as his or her needs, and therefore lead to action. Presumably, the tendency to identify with other persons depends on social cues—proximity, length of association, and so on—which in the environment of adaptation have been reliable cues to kinship or to in-group membership (see chapter 3). Badcock's argument seems to capture something about the subjective feeling involved in altruism, at least between close kin. Parents, for example, seem to really feel their children's needs as if they were their own. But it also raises questions of a theoretical nature about variations in self-representations. If self-representations are like umbrellas, which can expand or contract to cover in some functional sense surrounding groups or persons, then individual self-representations differ not only in self-efficacy, self-esteem, or resource holding power, but also in extent. Some selves may be more expansive than others, or selectively deficient. The schizoid's self-representation, for example, may differ from normal self-representations by not embracing the group. Extent of the self-representation may also determine self-efficacy. Certainly, resource holding power is in fact mostly determined by the extent to which individuals incorporate and coordinate their activities with others (see chapter 4). This would explain the collapse of self-efficacy, self-esteem, or RHP consequent on object loss in depressive patients.

The advantage of following up Badcock's lead is that the language of self-representations may provide a way of conceptualizing problems, or interpersonal differences, which patients might find useful. Self-representations can also be studied objectively.

Extended self-representations have been noted in observations on monozygotic twins, which are reviewed by Segal (1988). Many identical twin pairs report feeling closer to each other than to anyone else. They avoid separations and coordinate their activities. They experience themselves as parts of a single whole. Whatever the immediate causes of identification to this extreme degree, and it is easy to imagine what some of these might be, it makes inclusive fitness sense, and sense in Badcock's theory, that self-representations are sufficiently expansible to fully incorporate other individuals with identical genes.

Expectations of others, based on prior experience, also affect adherence to social strategies. In the course of growing up, individuals learn to expect certain behavioral patterns from those on whom they rely, from people with whom they compete, and from friends. Unfortunate social experiences—with an abusive parent, for instance—create expectations that lead to later problems in adherence to strategies. I noted in chapter 3 that modern attachment theorists account for stable patterns of separation behavior in terms of representations formed of attachment figures. Presumably, long-term problems related to childlike aid-seeking strategies also depend in part on this type of representation. Similar notions apply to competitive strategies and to reciprocal altruism. Psychodynamic therapies focus on expectations based on previous social experience, which are revealed in transference. I am referring to transference in its broader sense, as a reenactment of earlier relationships.

Expectations of others are tightly interwoven with self-representations. Estimates of resource holding power, for instance, are in large part determined by beliefs concerning the power, hostility, and unpredictability of other people.

Inhibitions and feelings of guilt also affect social strategies. I noted in chapter 4 that sexual strategies are subject to inhibitions. In an inclusive fitness sense, sexual inhibitions most likely serve the interests of others. Competitive and aid-seeking strategies are also especially vulnerable to inhibitions and guilt. Inhibitions and feelings of guilt are obviously dependent on prior social experience. They are conditions of love expressed by parents and other powerful figures in the child's life. They are therefore interwoven with representations of others and with self-regard. Psychodynamic therapies try to trace problematic inhibitions and feelings of guilt to their interpersonal roots and to supplant them with different codes of conduct.

A number of authors interested in the psychological implications of sociobiology have argued for the importance of self-deception (Alexander, 1975, 1979, 1987; Lockard, 1980; Trivers, 1974, 1981, 1985; see also, Badcock, 1986; Krebs, et al., 1988; Slavin, 1985). Several social strategies, especially reciprocal altruism and sexual competition, require individuals to hide from other persons selfish, aggressive, or even sexual motives. Since it is hard to avoid betraying knowledge of guilt, it might be adaptive to deceive oneself concerning one's own motives before attempting to deceive others. Thus, individuals who are capable of seeing themselves in a good light while acting on base motives might be more fit than those who see themselves more realistically. In this regard, studies purportedly show that mildly depressed individuals—whose self-esteem is generally rather poor (see chapter 3)—see themselves more realistically than do normal persons (see Krebs, et al., 1988)! Normal persons apparently maintain their self-esteem by viewing themselves selectively through rose colored glasses.

The sociobiological emphasis on deception and self-deception may seem to support Freudian conflict theory, according to which self-deceptive processes are pathogenic factors causing mental illness (Badcock, 1986; Fenichel, 1945). But though everyone may deceive himself, and though sociobiological models might show why self-deceptive perceptual biases are advantageous, no proof exists that self-deception plays an etiologic role in specific mental disorders, which is the crux of conflict theory. The issue is not whether people deceive themselves, but whether they fall ill because they deceive themselves. The findings noted above concerning depressive illness, together with sociobiological considerations concerning self-esteem, indicate that people might fall ill when they do not deceive themselves. Several studies review various types of evidence pertinent to assessment of Freudian conflict theory (Fisher and Greenberg, 1985; Greenberg and Mitchell, 1983; Mitchell, 1988).

All these psychological factors are greatly affected by superstitious and religious beliefs. Individuals who believe they have commerce with supernatural beings are likely to feel more or less powerful, more or less certain of others, and more or less in need of atonement as the result of their belief system. Superstitious and religious beliefs are in large part culturally determined, and consequently fall under the rubric of social factors affecting strategic functioning, but the sociobiological viewpoint suggests they are also generated *de novo* by psychological processes intrinsic to each individual. Thus, certain types of superstitious and religious notions would complicate mental functioning even in a society that appears to be wholly secular and discourages superstition. I will explain this assertion here, since it sheds additional light on the view of mental life implicit in the model adopted in this book. Sociobiological models suggest that beliefs in unseen beings play a wider role in psychological life than psychological theories have thus far acknowledged. Readers interested in a fuller discussion of the sociobiological psychology of religion are referred to my earlier work (Wenegrat, 1990).

In chapter 2 I noted that human cognitive processes were most likely shaped by social selective pressures, rather than by selective pressures by nonhuman forces. Spencer (1851), Darwin (1871), and Baldwin (1896) advanced this viewpoint in the nineteenth century, even before ethological and sociobiological studies demonstrated the intensity of social strategic pressures. More recently, Chance (1962) and Humphrey (1976) have restated the argument in more modern terms (see also Symons, 1987). According to Chance (1962), superior intellectual capacities conferred advantages in dealing with other minds. They produced increasingly complex social environments that exerted still stronger pressures in favor of greater intelligence. No such positive feedback loop could be formed with selective pressures outside the social arena. Humphrey (1976) argued that human intelligence is "dedicated" to playing certain social games. "Domain specific" is a more recent term denoting dedication of intellectual processes (see, for example, Cosmides and Tooby, 1989; Tooby and Cosmides, 1989). As I noted in chapter 2, computer equipment dedicated to a particular task is configured to achieve that task with maximal efficiency. It can achieve other tasks, or run other programs, but only with less efficiency, or in human terms, by expending greater effort.

Most recently, cognitive psychologists, too, have begun to note the importance of considering the adaptive social functions of human intellectual processes in order to avoid drawing invalid conclusions (see, for example, Cole, et al., 1982; Cooper, 1987; Cosmides and Tooby, 1987; Neisser, 1982; Wyer and Srull, 1984, 1986; see also Chomsky, 1980; Fodor, 1980, 1983). In this vein, Cosmides and Tooby (Cosmides, 1989; Cosmides and Tooby, 1989; Tooby and Cosmides, 1989) demonstrated that apparent logical errors elicited by certain tasks may be understood in light of the social origin of intellectual processes.

Social analytic skills needed for adherence to innately probable strategies were noted in previous chapters. As I observed in chapter 2, making adjustments for cultural norms, humans must categorize others as reliable or not, judge power relationships dependent on social-political networks, surmise hidden actors and intentions behind complex events, trace kinship relationships, imitate authority figures, see their own actions as they appear to others, calculate the responses others will likely make, and creatively compromise when interests are in conflict.

In a previous work I argued that social analytic skills produce beliefs in supernatural beings (Wenegrat, 1990). In particular, the tendency to surmise actors, intentions, and social interventions from complex events will lead to such beliefs when the events in question are outside the social realm. Since surmises of this type come readily to humans—who have been selected for the ease with which they make them—attempts to understand the natural world with the human mind inevitably lead to belief in unseen beings. For example, social events are instigated. When social analytic skills are applied to natural events, the result is inevitably belief in a hidden instigator. Social events have social meaning. When social analytic skills are applied to natural events, the result is inevitably an assignment of social meaning. Social events can be influenced. When social analytic skills are applied to natural events, the result is inevitably an attempt at social influence.

Supernatural beings play a prominent role in most religious systems, which attribute to them certain consensual features. In this way religions harness for social ends the individual's tendency to think in social terms. I noted in my earlier work that more idiosyncratic supernatural beings also play a prominent role in culturally disapproved superstitions, such as the Monte Carlo Fallacy, and in children's thinking (Wenegrat, 1990). Of course, many people are neither religious nor admit to superstitions, so it is easy to conclude that supernatural beings play no essential role in human mental life. That is, it is easy to conclude that human beings are capable of unalloyed rational thinking. This would be a mistake, though, since it fails to probe deeply enough into religious disbelief on the one hand and mental life on the other.

With regard to disbelief, intensive studies of atheists and agnostics indicate that religious disbelief is frequently ambiguous or superficial (see, for example, Allport and Ross, 1967; Hood, 1978; Rizzuto, 1976, 1979; Vergote, 1988; Vernon, 1968; Vitz, 1988). Freud (1907, 1913, 1927, 1939) believed that the image of God is based on that of the Oedipal father; empirical studies seem to show that the image of God incorporates attributes of both parents, and not just those of the father (Beit-Hallahmi and Argyle, 1975; Larsen and Knapp, 1964; Nelson, 1971; Nelson and Jones, 1957; Siegman, 1961; Strunk, 1959; Vergote, et al., 1969). In any event, studies show that many apparent atheists or agnostics imagine a god figure resembling a parent toward whom they have ambivalent feelings. They defy their parental god by skepticism or disbelief (see, for example, Rizzuto, 1979). In other cases, atheists or agnostics have rejected parental religions as a way of defying their parents, and not for the rational reasons they cite for their decision.

With regard to mental life, a clue to the hidden importance of imagined unseen agents is found in Freud's treatment of superstition, compulsion, and the Superego. In *The Psychopathology of Everyday Life,* Freud (1901) described superstition as the expectation of trouble, based on the fear of retribution for repressed hostile wishes. Fear of retribution, of course, imples belief in an unseen punitive agent. Later, Freud (1923) named the agent that individuals fear the Superego, and he suggested that, like the image of God, it is formed from models provided by the parents. Freud's writings imply that he thought of the Superego as a privately worshipped god. For example, Freud (1907, also 1919) had earlier argued that obsessional neuroses are "private religious system(s)" and religion a "universal obsessional neurosis." Obsessional rituals play in the private religion the same role liturgy plays in the public neurosis. But after inventing his structural theory, Freud (1923) argued, without retracting his earlier formulation, that compulsion neuroses are aimed at appeasing the Superego (see also Fenichel, 1945). Consequently, insofar as obsessional neuroses are still to be considered private religions, the Superego must be the object of private worship, or a private god. And, insofar as religion is still to be considered a public obsessional neurosis, God must be a consensual Superego!

The German term "Ich," rendered into "ego" by Freud's English translators, literally mean the "I" (Bettelheim, 1982; Brandt, 1966; see also Eagle, 1984). "Uber-Ich," rendered into "superego," refers to a functional agency somehow "above-the-I." What better name could Freud have found for a functioning private god?

Observers of modern culture (see, for example, Rieff, 1966) have noted the extent to which psychoanalysts and psychotherapists have assumed what were previously priestly functions. This is especially the case insofar as therapists deal with guilt and try to define just repentance; in other words, insofar as they try to intercede between the individual and his Superego, or his private god. Apparently, individuals applying social analytic schemata to their circumstances render unto the resulting deities that which they think is owed them. Public, explicit appeasement is in the domain of religion. If intercession is needed, a priest will be consulted. Private, implicit appeasement is in the domain of analysis. If intercession is needed, a psychotherapist will be consulted.

What this argument suggests, or course, is that people lead their social lives not only in relation to real and past others, as object-relational theories suppose, but also in relation to hypostasized beings who are continually recreated by social cognitive processes, characteristic of humans, applied to the world at large. These beings are interpreted in conventional terms, and in terms of past relationships, and may or may not be acknowledged in a public arena. Insofar as they become conscious they may be subjected to more critical scrutiny, but they are unlikely to ever entirely lose their force. They comprise an important factor complicating behavior of human beings.

Several types of social conditions affect adherence to strategies. First there are conditions of a less personal type. These include religion, cultural norms, economic circumstance, and technological factors.

I have already mentioned inhibitions and feelings of guilt. These are clearly dependent on religious and moral beliefs inculcated in children in particular groups. I have elsewhere summarized social strategic aspects of religious beliefs (Wenegrat, 1990).

Secular cultural norms affect adherence to social strategies in a pervasive way. For many Americans, for instance, the ideal adult is independent, competitive, and uninvolved in social groups (see Bellah, et al., 1985). People with this ideal suppress desires for aid, cultivate aggressiveness, and inhibit wishes to belong to close-knit groups. Childlike strategies aimed at obtaining aid, competitive strategies, and strategies relating to groups are consequently affected. Certain other societies promote the opposite virtues, with opposite social effects (see, for example, Erikson, 1963).

Social class is also very important. In the United States, social class determines how well children are cared for, and consequently the fate of childhood social strategies. In adulthood, social class dictates competitive options and helps to shape feelings about the group as a whole. Virtually every strategy is altered in some way by constraints that vary with social class. Major improvements in mental health in the United States will never be achieved without first ameliorating the destructive effects wrought by extreme social class differences in stresses and opportunities.

I noted in chapter 4 that the apparent economic emancipation of women now slowly occurring in Western countries may signify a return to cultural patterns in which women control resources needed for raising children. A cultural change of this type should have important effects on psychological functioning and on mental health, since, as I observed in chapter 4, when women control resources needed for raising children, they are likely to shift to a different reproductive strategy than when they depend on men. They are likely to be less sexually inhibited and to prefer nonexclusive relationships. This is because they no longer need to trade paternity confidence for male-controlled resources. Men may even drain child-rearing resources under certain conditions, and in these situations women may prefer to avoid becoming involved with them for more than sexual liaisons. With changes in female strategies, male intra-sex competition may greatly diminish and be shifted from the arena of resource accumulation.

I noted in chapter 4 that in many societies parents use sexual ideologies to ensure that their daughters adhere to a sexually inhibited, male-dependent reproductive strategy. By indoctrinating their daughters to avoid sexual intercourse except when it is sanctioned, parents protect them from men who will not provide for their children. They also ensure that their daughters will be willing to give their husbands confidence of paternity in exchange for aid. Inclusive fitness considerations suggest that if women come to control resources needed for rearing children, parents will be less apt to impart stringent mores concerning sexual matters. Ideologic change consequent on altered parental inclusive fitness interests may even precede changes in female reproductive strategies induced by economic circumstances, and play a causal role in them. In any event, ideologic change can be expected to reduce the frequency of sexual inhibitions in both men and women, together with the adverse effects these have on mental health.

Alterations in female mating strategies might also have effects on specific syndromes. As I described in chapter 4, Draper and Harpending (1988) argued that sociopathic and hysterical personality traits manifest an underlying disposition to cheat in male and female reproductive strategies, respectively. The sociopathic male cheats by deceiving women; the hysterical female cheats by deceiving men. But men have a harder time cheating women who do not need them. And likewise, independent women have no reason to seek any male assistance. So both sociopathic traits in men and hysterical traits in women might be rendered pointless if women controlled resources needed for rearing children. In this regard, it is interesting to note that the heyday of female hysteria was in the last century, when there were few if any opportunities for independent women. The female hysterics described by Charcot were sexually abused, poverty-stricken, and desperate. They needed assistance from others even to survive (see Drinka, 1984).

When fathers are no longer essential to child-rearing, their role in the family structure—if the family as we know it exists—will be greatly modified. Parental interactions will be more democratic and less patriarchal, and there will be fewer opportunities for male violence in the family than there are at present. Fathers will earn their keep in the family by their nurturant, friendly, and supportive behavior rather than just by bringing food to the table. I noted in chapter 4 that boys may learn how to deal with intrasex competition from early interactions with their fathers. Numerous studies have shown that friendly and supportive paternal behavior causes boys to identify with other men (see Fisher and Greenberg, 1985) and to be less aggressive (cf. Guidubaldi, et al., 1983; Hetherington, 1979; Hodges and Bloom, 1984; Hodges, et al., 1983). In egalitarian families, girls may be better protected against paternal sexual abuse than they have been in the past, which may make for significant changes in female mental health.

On the other hand, the extremely high divorce rate in our society seems, in terms of the models developed in this book, a sign that men today are victimizing women and children by pursuing their sexual strategy—to optimize access to reproductive potential—without the societal sanctions that previously restrained them (see Mac-Donald, 1988c; Mackey, 1980). That the benefits of divorce are unequally shared in our society is illustrated by the fact that divorced women and their children, but not divorced men, comprise a growing segment of those living in poverty (see Hetherington, 1979; Wallerstein and Kelly, 1980). Also, divorced men, but not divorced women, are likely to remarry and to start new families (Mackey, 1980). Apparently, male-controlled resources are being used in many cases to create new families at the expense of old ones. There are also numerous studies showing how children suffer in our society following a divorce, in ways that are likely to inflict permanent harm (Guidubaldi, et al., 1983; Hetherington, 1972, 1979; Hodges and Bloom, 1984; Hodges, et al., 1983; Wallerstein and Kelly, 1980). Of course, I do not mean to imply that, in seeking divorces, men are thinking in terms of inclusive fitness. Only a miniscule fraction of divorced men know what inclusive fitness is, much less how to estimate how their behavior affects it. Instead, men have evolved to desire multiple partners and to more readily depreciate children's interests. Consequently, serial monogamy, which is what our divorce laws make possible, is more attractive to men than to women, at least in our society. Divorce could only be even-handed in a society where women really controlled access to equal resources.

In chapter 4 I described Draper and Harpending's (1982, 1988) theory, that absence of the father serves as a discriminant cue for alternative female reproductive strategies. According to Draper and Harpending, girls raised without a father present will pursue a reproductive strategy without regard for male parental investment. Consequently, the increased frequency of divorce in our society might hasten the transition toward female independence due to a changing female role in the economy.

Technological factors affect social strategies in unpredictable ways; some effects become obvious only retrospectively. For example, obstetric medical practices may disrupt maternal-infant interactions during a "critical period" shortly after birth. Disrupted interactions might lead to later changes in maternal care and therefore in childhood strategies aimed at obtaining aid (see, for example, Ali and Lowry, 1981; DeChateau and Wiberg, 1977a, 1977b; Hales, et al., 1977; Trowell, 1982). For this reason, obstetricians and nurses currently make an effort to preserve interactions between mothers and infants. Technologically stimulated changes in feeding practices (see, for example, Knoedel, 1977) might also affect relationships between mothers and infants and consequently alter later strategic activity. This is an area about which little is known.

Effective contraceptive techniques might alter sexual strategies in the same way as female resource control. Even women dependent on male child-rearing assistance might be freed by contraceptive techniques to engage in coital relations with men they will not marry, without risking reduced inclusive fitness. By diminishing the risk of pregnancy, these same techniques decrease parents' incentives to indoctrinate their daughters. Contraception, therefore, might alleviate psychological problems created by sexual mores protecting parental interests. However, whether female sexual strategies, and parental behaviors, will really shift because of contraceptive techniques depends on whether these techniques affect evolved contingent cues concerning resource needs, such as the one suggested by Draper and Harpending (1982, 1988), which presumably control female reproductive strategies. Other than long-term nursing, effective means for preventing impregnation were presumably not practiced in the environment in which humans evolved; they cannot, consequently, be contingent cues themselves. If they affect only some evolved contingent cues, and not others, contraceptive techniques may induce only a partial strategic shift, in comparison with shifts induced by female resource control. Or contraceptive techniques may affect reproductive strategies by permitting women to play a different role in the economy, thereby helping them to gain resource control.

To give another example, new means of travel have important effects on strategies relating to social groups. Mass transit and automobiles allow individuals to work far from their homes. Modern suburbs are sometimes called "bedroom communities," implying they are not communities in a more general sense. The same technological factors allow people to leave their communities altogether by moving readily to different cities or states. On the other hand mass culture insures that when they arrive, their environment will not seem totally unfamiliar.

Other technological factors affecting particular strategies readily come to mind, once we start thinking in these terms.

More personal social conditions also have effects on adherence to various strategies. First, personal history—especially experience with parents and other family—obviously determines much of social development. Self-representations and expectations of others both seem to be forged from early social experience. I have already shown how these might affect later social behaviors related to competitive and childlike aid-seeking strategies. I have also seen cases in which early peer relations, or experiences with parents who themselves were alienated, have affected later strategies relating to social groups. Good experiences with peer groups may ameliorate the effects of alienated parents.

It is common clinical experience that many patients do not know their own personal history, or at least important details, in spite of the fact that they show effects in their social behavior. By reconstructing patients' personal histories, psychotherapists may lay the cognitive basis for later behavioral change.

Present personal circumstances is also clearly important in social strategic terms. Recent losses, for instance, are likely to stimulate strategies aimed at obtaining aid. Recent failures are likely to alter self-efficacy, especially if self-efficacy is tenuous or unstable. Changes in self-efficacy will lead to changes in strategies aimed at obtaining aid and in competitive strategies. I have shown elsewhere how various social disruptions, such as those that occur when young people go to college, can lead to important changes in manifestations of strategies relating to social groups (Wenegrat, 1989). Clinicians of all stripes are very highly attuned to the role of recent events in triggering mental disorders.

In general, patients interpret events according to the strategies that are most salient for them. Ill health, for instance, may pose a threat to security, to status, or to membership in the social group, depending on whether the ill patient is more preoccupied with aid-seeking, competitive, or group-related strategies. How patients interpret events like physical illness provides important clues to their salient social strategies.

To summarize, the sociobiological framework developed in previous chapters encompasses factors of many different types affecting social behavior. Biological, psychological, and past and present social factors are all considered possible causes of mental disorder. Any of these factors that potentially can be remedied should be targets of therapy. By altering one or more remediable factors producing strategic dysfunction, the clinician might be able to shift strategic functioning in the direction of health.

The Psychotherapist as an Authority Figure

In his famous book, *Persuasion and Healing,* Frank (1974) argued that powerful curative factors are mobilized by social groups acting through designated authorities in healing arts, and that these are not dependent on technical interventions. Numerous empirical studies support Frank's argument; they attest to the curative powers of group authority figures lacking effective technologies (see, for example, the classic work by McCardel and Murray, 1974; also Finkelstein, et al., 1982; Frances, et al., 1985). Our own society designates psychiatrists, psychologists, and certain other therapists as authorities empowered to heal mental disorders. As I noted earlier, many authors have observed that therapists today perform the functions once served by priests and ministers. I noted one way in which the roles played by therapists and priests overlap. They also overlap in that both therapists and priests are designated authorities who bring consensual systems to bear on personal problems. That the systems used by therapists and priests differ is probably less important than that they are both consensual.

Many psychotherapists find the notion that they are instruments of the social group rather uncongenial; in fact, many therapists see themselves as helping the patient resist past and present pressures imposed by other persons. Other therapists see themselves as helping the patient address existential issues that are inherently private. Yet, psychotherapists are trained in institutions accredited and licensed by public organizations. They are licensed by the state, have their offices in public places, and advertise themselves as members of a profession. The mere fact that they are perceived as successfully making their living by treating other persons makes psychotherapists into public personae, who have a place in the social group acknowledged by those who pay them.

The sociobiological models described in chapter 4 provide a theoretical basis for interpreting Frank's observation. These models indicate that in order to adhere to mutualistic and reciprocal altruistic social strategies, humans evolved powerful affective, cognitive, and perceptual dispositions that cause them to cling to social groups and to adopt their thinking.

There are a number of ways in which psychotherapists employ group social power to promote improved functioning. First, all psychotherapists to some extent use suggestion. If nothing else, they suggest to their patients that relief will result from following certain treatment procedures. As a type of conformity, suggestion must manifest cognitive dispositions leading to group adhesion. To the extent that the therapist is seen as the embodiment of objective, or group, reality, his or her suggestions will carry greater force.

Second, therapists often must induce their patients to change their cognitive models or their style of living. They do so by convincing patients that their models of themselves, of others, or of their circumstances are different from the models others would construct on the basis of adequate data. They convince patients, in other words, that their cognitive models are out of conformity with those that would be consensual if the group somehow knew what the therapist knows about them. In this process, the therapist is implicitly speaking for other people, who presumably would agree with the therapist if they were actually present in the therapy sessions. But the therapist, of course, can speak for other people only insofar as he or she is an authority figure empowered to convey reality to patients.

Finally, individuals who fail to adhere to innately probable strategies, or who pursue these strategies in an aberrant form, are alienated to that extent from their social group. They inevitably perceive that they are somehow different from the normative models offered by the group. In chapter 4, I mentioned studies that appear to show that alienation produces affective distress, which is relieved following integration into a social group. The same type of distress might compound the problems of those who see that they have psychological problems. By placing psychological problems, and failures to conform to normative life patterns, in a consensual framework, the therapist symbolically ushers the patient back into the social group. Group therapy methods can also overcome alienation of those with mental disorders, in this case by creating a microcosm. To symbolically usher the patient back into the social group, the therapist relies on his or her public mandate to speak for the group at large.

Insofar as psychotherapeutic treatment effects depend on the higher-order social setting in which therapy occurs, rather than on specific technical interventions or on the dyadic relationship, prognosis should be better for patients who can readily integrate themselves into a social group. The difficulties encountered in treating schizoid or schizotypal patients, for example, may be due to their failure to respond to cognitive authority figures or to conform with consensual reality. The social strategy that must, so to speak, carry the burden of cure is dysfunctional in these cases. In chapter 4, I noted that therapists who are most successful in treating schizotypal and schizophrenic patients are those who voice reality—as it appears to most people—in the clearest possible way.

Bibliography

Abraham, K. 1927. Notes on the psycho-analytical investigation and treatment of manic-depressive insanity and related conditions. In *Selected Papers of Karl Abraham,* London: Hogarth Press.

Abrams, R., and Taylor, M.A. 1974. Unipolar and bipolar depressive illness: Phenomenology and response to ECT. *Archives of General Psychiatry* 30:320.

————. 1980. A comparison of unipolar and bipolar depressive illness. *American Journal of Psychiatry* 137:1084.

Abrahamson, L.Y., Metalsky, G.I., and Alloy, L.B. 1989. Hopelessness depression: A theory-based subtype of depression. *Psychological Review* 96:358.

Abrahamson, L.Y., Seligman, M.E.P., and Teasdale, J.D. 1978. Learned helplessness in humans: Critique and reformulation. *Journal of Abnormal Psychology* 87:49.

Adams, N.S., and Neel, J.V. 1967. Children of incest. *Pediatrics* 40:50.

Adler, G. 1979. The myth of the alliance with borderline patients. *American Journal of Psychiatry* 136:642.

Adorno, T.W., Frenkel-Brunswick, E., Levinson, D.J., et al. 1950. *The Authoritarian Personality.* New York: Harper and Brother.

Agren, G. 1984. Incest avoidance and bonding between siblings in gerbils. *Behavioral Ecology and Sociobiology* 14:161.

Ainsworth, M.D. 1963. The development of infant-mother interaction among the Ganda. In *Determinants of Infant Behaviour,* Vol. 2. B.M. Foss, editor. London: Methuen.

————. 1982. Attachment: Retrospect and prospect. In *The Place of Attachment in Human Behavior.* C.M. Parkes, and J. Stevenson-Hinde, editors. New York: Basic Books.

Ainsworth, M.D., Blehar, M.C., Waters, E., et al. 1978. *Patterns of Attachment: A Psychological Study of the Strange Situation.* Hillsdale, N.J.: Erlbaum.

Ainsworth, M.D., and Wittig, B.A. 1969. Attachment and the exploratory behavior of one-year-olds in a strange situation. In *Determinants of Infant Behaviour,* Vol. 4. B.M. Foss, editor. London: Methuen.

Akhtar, S., and Byrne, J.P. 1983. The concept of splitting and its clinical relevance. *American Journal of Psychiatry* 140:1013.

Akiskal, H.S. 1981. Subaffective disorders: Dysthymic, cyclothymic and bipolar II disorders in the "borderline" realm. *Psychiatric Clinics of North America* 4:25.

Akiskal, H.S., Dijenderdjian, A.H., Rosenthal, R.H., et al. 1977. Cyclothymic disorder: Validating criteria for inclusion in the bipolar affective group. *American Journal of Psychiatry* 134:1227.

Akiskal, H.S., and McKinney, W.T. Jr. 1975. Overview of recent research in depression: Integration of ten conceptual models into a comprehensive clinical frame. *Archives of General Psychiatry* 32:285.

Alexander, R.D. 1974. The evolution of social behavior. *Annual Review of Ecology and Systematics* 5:325.

———. 1975. The search for a general theory of behavior. *Behavior Science* 20:77.

———. 1979. *Darwinism and Human Affairs.* Seattle: University of Washington Press.

———. 1987. *The Biology of Moral Systems.* New York: Aldine De Gruyter.

Alexander, R.D., Hoogland, J.L., Howard, R.D., et al. 1979. Sexual dimorphisms and breeding systems in pinnipeds, ungulates, primates, and humans. In *Evolutionary Biology and Human Social Behavior: An Anthropological Perspective.* N.A. Chagnon, and W. Irons, editors. North Scituate, MA: Duxbury Press.

Ali, Z., and Lowry, M. 1981. Early maternal-child contact: Effects on later behaviour. *Developmental Medicine and Child Neurology* 23:337.

Allen, R.O., and Spilka, B. 1967. Committed and consensual religion: A specification of religion-prejudice relationships. *Journal for the Scientific Study of Religion* 6:191.

Allodi, F. 1982. Acute paranoid reaction (Boufee Delirante) in Canada. *Canadian Journal of Psychiatry* 27:366.

Allport, G.W. 1966. The religious context of prejudice. *Journal for the Scientific Study of Religion* 5:447.

Allport, G.W., and Ross, J.M. 1967. Personal religious orientation and prejudice. *Journal of Personality and Social Psychology* 5:432.

Altmann, S.A., and Altmann, J. 1970. *Baboon Ecology: African Field Research.* Chicago: University of Chicago Press.

American Psychiatric Association 1987. *Diagnostic and Statistical Manual of Mental Disorders,* 3rd Ed., revised. Washington, D.C.: American Psychiatric Press.

Anderson, B.S., and Zinsser, J.P. 1988. *A History of Their Own: Women in Europe from Prehistory to the Present.* New York: Harper and Row.

Andrulonis, P.A., Glueck, B.L., Stroebel, C.F., et al. 1981. Organic brain dysfunction and the borderline syndrome. *Psychiatric Clinics of North America* 4:47.

Anstadt, T., and Krause, R. 1989. The expression of primary affects in portraits drawn by schizophrenics. *Psychiatry* 52:13.

Anthony, E.J. 1968. The developmental precursors of adult schizophrenia. *Journal of Psychiatric Research* 6:293.

Aoki, K. 1986. A stochastic model of gene-culture coevolution suggested by the "culture historical hypothesis" for the evolution of adult lactose absorption in humans. *Proceedings of the National Academy of Sciences of the United States of America* 83:2929.

Arend, R., Gove, F., and Sroufe, L.A. 1979. Continuity of individual adaptation from infancy to kindergarten: A predictive study of ego-resiliency and curiosity in pre-schoolers. *Child Development* 50:950.

Arieti, S., and Bemporad, J. 1978. *Severe and Mild Depression: The Psychotherapeutic Approach.* New York: Basic Books.

———. 1980. The psychological organization of depression. *American Journal of Psychiatry* 137:1360.

Arling, G.L., and Harlow, H.F. 1967. Effects of social deprivation on maternal behavior of rhesus monkeys. *Journal of Comparative and Physiological Psychology* 64:371.

Arrindell, W.A., Emmelkamp, P.M.G., Monsma, A., et al. 1983. Perceived parental rearing practices in phobic disorders. *British Journal of Psychiatry* 143: 183.

Asch, S.E. 1956. Studies of independence and conformity: I. A minority of one against a unanimous majority. *Psychological Monographs* 70(9):1.

Audy, J.R. 1980. Man the lonely animal: Biological roots of loneliness. In *The Anatomy of Loneliness.* J. Hartog, J.R. Audy, and Y.A. Cohen, editors. New York: International Universities Press.

Axelrod, R. 1984. *The Evolution of Cooperation.* New York: Basic Books.

Axelrod, R., and Hamilton, W.D. 1981. The evolution of cooperation. *Science* 211:1390.

Badcock, C.R. 1986. *The Problem of Altruism: Freudian-Darwinian Solutions.* New York: Basil Blackwell.

Baldwin, J.M. 1896. A new factor in evolution. *American Naturalist* 30:441.

———. 1897. *Social and Ethical Interpretations in Mental Development: A Study in Social Psychology.* New York: MacMillan.

Ballenger, J.C. 1988. Biological aspects of depression: Implications for clinical practice. In *American Psychiatric Press Review of Psychiatry,* Vol. 7. A.J. Frances, and R.E. Hales, eds. Washington, D.C.: American Psychiatric Press.

Bandura, A. 1977. Self-efficacy: Toward a unifying theory of behavioral change. *Psychological Review* 84:191.

———. 1986. *Social Foundations of Thought and Action: A Social Cognitive Theory.* Englewood Cliffs, NJ: Prentice-Hall.

Bandura, A., Adams, N.E., and Beyer, J. 1977. Cognitive processes mediating behavioral change. *Journal of Personality and Social Psychology* 35:125.

Barash, D. 1979. *Sociobiology: The Whisperings Within.* New York: Harper and Row.

———. 1982. *Sociobiology and Behavior,* 2nd ed. New York: Elsevier.

Barkow, J.H. 1989. The elastic between genes and culture. *Ethology and Sociobiology* 10:111.

Barlow, D.H. 1988. Current models of panic disorder and a view from emotion theory. In *American Psychiatric Press Review of Psychiatry,* Vol. 7. A.J. Frances, and R.E. Hales, eds. Washington, D.C.: American Psychiatric Press.

Baron, M., Gruen, R., Asnis, E., et al. 1983. Familial relatedness of schizophrenia and schizotypal states. *American Journal of Psychiatry* 140:1437.

Baron, M., Klotz, J., Mendlewicz, J., et al. 1981. Multiple-threshold transmission of affective disorders. *Archives of General Psychiatry* 38:79.

Barrash, I., Kroll, J., Carey, K., et al. 1983. Discriminating borderline disorder from other personality disorders: Cluster analysis of the diagnostic interview for borderlines. *Archives of General Psychiatry* 40:1297.

Bateson, P. 1978. Sexual imprinting and optimal outbreeding. *Nature* 273:659.

———. 1982. Behavioral development and evolutionary processes. In *Current Problems in Sociobiology.* King's College Sociobiology Group, editors. Cambridge: Cambridge University Press.

Beardslee, W.R., Bemporad, J., Keller, M.B., et al. 1983. Children of parents with major affective disorder: A review. *American Journal of Psychiatry* 140:825.

Bebbington, P.E., Brugha, T., MacCarthy, B., et al. 1988. The Camberwell collaborative depression study. I. Depressed probands: Adversity and the form of depression. *British Journal of Psychiatry* 152:754.

Beck, A.T. 1972. *Depression: Causes and Treatment.* Philadelphia: University of Pennsylvania Press.

———. 1976. *Cognitive Therapy and the Emotional Disorders.* New York: International Universities Press.

Beck, A.T., Weissman, A., Lester, D., et al. 1974. The measurement of pessimism. *Journal of Consulting and Clinical Psychology* 42:861.

Beit-Hallahmi, B., and Argyle, M. 1975. God as a father-projection: The theory and the evidence. *British Journal of Medical Psychology* 48:71.

Bell, A.P., and Weinberg, M.S. 1978. *Homosexualities: A Study of Diversity among Men and Women.* New York: Simon and Schuster.

Bell, A.P., Weinberg, M.S., and Hammersmith, S.K. 1981. *Sexual Preference: Its Development in Men and Women.* Bloomington: Indiana University Press.

Bell, J., Lycaki, H., Jones, D., et al. 1983. Effect of pre-existing borderline personality disorder on clinical and EEG sleep correlates of depression. *Psychiatry Research* 9:115.

Bellah, R.N., Madsen, R., Sullivan, W.M., et al. 1985. *Habits of the Heart: Individualism and Commitment in American Life.* Berkeley: University of California Press.

Belsky, J., Rovine, M., and Taylor, D.G. 1984. The Pennsylvania infant and family development project, 3: The origins of individual differences in infant-mother attachment: Maternal and infant contributions. *Child Development* 55:718.

Berg, I. 1976. School phobia in the children of agoraphobic women. *British Journal of Psychiatry* 128:86.

Berg, I., Marks, I., McGuire, R., et al. 1974. School phobia and agoraphobia. *Psychological Medicine* 4:428.

Berger, P.A., and Brodie, H.K.H., eds. 1986. *American Handbook of Psychiatry,*

2nd ed., Vol. 8, *Biological Psychiatry.* New York: Basic Books.

Berger, P.L., and Luckmann, T. 1966. *The Social Construction of Reality: A Treatise in the Sociology of Knowledge.* Garden City, NJ: Doubleday.

Berkowitz, L. 1954. Group standards, cohesiveness, and productivity. *Human Relations* 7:509.

Berman, K.F., Illowsky, B.P., and Weinberger, D.R. 1988. Physiological dysfunction of dorsolateral prefrontal cortex in schizophrenia. IV. Further evidence for regional and behavioral specificity. *Archives of General Psychiatry* 45:616.

Bertram, B.C.R. 1982. Problems with altruism. In *Current Problems in Sociobiology.* King's College Sociobiology Group, editors. Cambridge: Cambridge University Press.

Bettelheim, B. 1982. *Freud and Man's Soul.* New York: Knopf.

Billig, M., and Tajfel, H. 1973. Social categorization and similarity in intergroup behaviour. *European Journal of Social Psychology* 3:27.

Binswanger, L. 1958. The case of Ellen West: An anthropological-clinical study. In *Existence.* R. May, E. Angel, and H.F. Ellenberger, editors. New York: Simon and Schuster.

Birtchnell, J. 1988. Depression and family relationships: A study of young, married women on a London housing estate. *British Journal of Psychiatry* 153:758.

Bishop, D.T., Cannings, C., and Maynard Smith, J. 1978. The war of attrition with random rewards. *Journal of Theoretical Biology* 74:377.

Blain, J., and Barkow, J. 1988. Father involvement, reproductive strategies, and the sensitive period. In *Sociobiological Perspectives on Human Development.* K.B. MacDonald, ed. New York: Springer-Verlag.

Blanck, G., and Blanck, R. 1974. *Ego Psychology: Theory and Practice.* New York: Columbia University Press.

Blatt, S.J. 1974. Levels of object representation in anaclitic and introjective depression. *Psychoanalytic Study of the Child* 29:107.

Blatt, S.J., Quinlan, D.M., Chevron, E.S., et al. 1982. Dependency and self-criticism: Psychological dimensions of depression. *Journal of Consulting and Clinical Psychology* 50:113.

Blatt, S.J., and Schichman, 1983. Two primary configurations of psychopathology. *Psychoanalysis and Contemporary Thought* 6:187.

Blaustein, A.R. 1983. Kin recognition mechanisms: Phenotype matching or recognition alleles? *American Naturalist* 121:749.

Bleich, A., Siegel, B., Garb, R., et al. 1986. Post-traumatic stress disorder following combat exposure: Clinical features and psychopharmacological treatment. *British Journal of Psychiatry* 149:365.

Blick, J. 1977. Selection for traits which lower individual reproduction. *Journal of Theoretical Biology* 67:597.

Blumer, D., and Benson, D.F. 1975. Personality changes with frontal and temporal lobe lesions. In *Psychiatric Aspects of Neurologic Disease.* D.F. Benson, and D. Blumer, editors. New York: Grune and Stratton.

Blumer, D., and Heilbronn, M. 1981. The pain-prone disorder: A clinical and psychological profile. *Psychosomatics* 22:395.

Bock, K. 1980. *Human Nature and History: A Response to Sociobiology.* New York: Columbia University Press.

Bower, T.G.R. 1974. *Development in Infancy.* San Francisco: W.H. Freeman.

Bowlby, J. 1958. The nature of the child's tie to his mother. *International Journal of Psycho-Analysis* 39:350.

———. 1969. *Attachment and Loss:* Volume I. New York: Basic Books.

———. 1973. *Attachment and Loss:* Volume II. New York: Basic Books.

———. 1977. The making and breaking of affectional bonds, I: Aetiology and psychopathology in the light of attachment theory. *British Journal of Psychiatry* 130:201.

———. 1980. *Attachment and Loss:* Volume III. New York: Basic Books.

Boyd, J.H., Burke, J.D., Gruenberg, E., et al. 1984. Exclusion criteria of DSM-III: A study of co-occurrence of hierarchy-free syndromes. *Archives of General Psychiatry* 41:983.

Boyd, R., and Richerson, P.J. 1985. *Culture and the Evolutionary Process.* Chicago: University of Chicago Press.

Bradley, S.J. 1979. The relationship of early maternal separation to borderline personality in children and adolescents: A pilot study. *American Journal of Psychiatry* 136:424.

Brandt, E.M., Stevens, C.W., and Mitchell, G. 1971. Visual and social communication in adult isolate-reared monkeys. *Primates* 12:105.

Brandt, L.W. 1966. Process or structure? *Psychoanalytic Review* 53:50.

Brazelton, T., Tronick, E., Adamson, L., et al. 1975. Early mother-infant reciprocity. *Ciba Foundation Symposium* 33:137.

Breier, A., Charney, D.S., and Heninger, G.R. 1985. The diagnostic validity of anxiety disorders and their relationship to depressive illness. *American Journal of Psychiatry* 142:787.

Breier, A., Kelsoe, J.R., Kirwin, P.D., et al. 1988. Early parental loss and development of adult psychopathology. *Archives of General Psychiatry* 45:987.

Brenner, C. 1939. On the genesis of a case of paranoid dementia precox. *Journal of Nervous and Mental Disease* 90:483.

———. 1974. *An Elementary Textbook of Psychoanalysis,* Rev. Ed. Garden City, NJ: Anchor Books.

Bretherton, I. 1985. Attachment theory: Retrospect and prospect. *Monographs of the Society for Research in Child Development* 50(1–2):3.

Breuer, G. 1982. *Sociobiology and the Human Dimension.* Cambridge: Cambridge University Press.

Brewer, M.B., and Silver, M. 1978. In-group bias as a function of task characteristics. *European Journal of Social Psychology* 8:393.

Brockington, I.F., Altman, E., Hillier, V., et al. 1982. The clinical picture of bipolar affective disorder in its depressed phase: A report from London and Chicago. *British Journal of Psychiatry* 141:558.

Bronson, G.W. 1972. Infants' reactions to unfamiliar persons and novel objects. *Monographs of the Society for Research in Child Development* 37(3):1.

Brothers, L. 1989. A biological perspective on empathy. *American Journal of Psychiatry* 146:10.

Brown, G.W. 1982. Early loss and depression. In *The Place of Attachment in Human Behavior.* C.M. Parkes, and J. Stevenson-Hinde, editors. New York: Basic Books.

Brown, G.W., and Harris, T.O. 1978. *The Social Origins of Depression: A Study of Psychiatric Disorder in Women.* London: Tavistock.

Brown, G.W., Harris, T.O., and Copeland, J.R. 1977. Depression and loss. *British Journal of Psychiatry* 130:1.

Bryer, J.B., Nelson, B.A., Miller, J.B., et al. 1987. Childhood sexual and physical abuse as factors in adult psychiatric illness. *American Journal of Psychiatry* 144:1426.

Buck, R. 1976. *Human Motivation and Emotion.* New York: Wiley.

———. 1984. *The Communication of Emotion.* New York: Guilford.

Buglass, D., Clarke, J., Henderson, A.S., et al. 1977. A study of agoraphobic housewives. *Psychological Medicine* 7:73.

Bullough, V.L., and Bullough, B. 1977. *Sin, Sickness, and Sanity: A History of Sexual Attitudes.* New York: Meridian.

Burbank, V.K. 1987. Female aggression in cross-cultural perspective. *Behavior Science Research* 21:70.

Buskirk, R.E. 1975. Coloniality, activity patterns and feeding in a tropical orb-weaving spider. *Ecology* 56:1314.

Buss, D.M. 1984. Evolutionary biology and personality psychology: Toward a conception of human nature and individual differences. *American Psychologist* 39:1135.

———. 1987. Sex differences in human mate selection criteria: An evolutionary perspective. In *Sociobiology and Psychology: Ideas, Issues and Applications.* C. Crawford, M. Smith, and D. Krebs, eds. Hillsdale, NJ: Lawrence Erlbaum.

———. 1989. Sex differences in human mate preferences: Evolutionary hypotheses tested in 37 cultures. *Behavioral and Brain Sciences* 12:1.

Butter, C.M., Snyder, D.R., and McDonald, J.A. 1970. Effects of orbital frontal lesions on aversive and aggressive behaviors in rhesus monkeys. *Journal of Comparative and Physiological Psychology* 72:132.

Cahan, E. 1984. The genetic psychologies of James Mark Baldwin and Jean Piaget. *Developmental Psychology* 20:128.

Campbell, D.T. 1960. Blind variation and selective retention in creative thought as in other knowledge processes. *Psychological Review* 67:380.

———. 1978. Social morality norms as evidence of conflict between biological human nature and social system requirements. In *Morality as a Biological Phenomenon.* G.S. Stent, editor. Berlin: Dahlem Konferenzen.

Campos, J., and Stenberg, C. 1980. Perception of appraisal and emotion: The onset of social referencing. In *Infant Social Cognition.* M.E. Lamb, and L. Sherrod, editors. Hillsdale, NJ: Erlbaum.

Cannon, W.B. 1942. Voodoo death. *American Anthropologist* 44:169.

Caplan, A.L., ed. 1978. *The Sociobiology Debate: Readings on Ethical and Scientific Issues.* New York: Harper and Row.

Capstick, N. 1971. Chlorimipramine in obsessional states. *Psychosomatics* 12:322.

Carey, G. 1982. Genetic influences on anxiety neurosis and agoraphobia. In *The Biology of Anxiety.* R.J. Mathew, editor. New York: Brunner/Mazel.

Carlsson, S.G., Fagerberg, H., Horneman, G., et al. 1978. Effects of amount of contact between mother and child on the mother's nursing behavior. *Developmental Psychobiology* 11:143.

Carroll, B.J., Greden, J.T., Feinberg, M., et al. 1981. Neuroendocrine evaluation of depression in borderline patients. *Psychiatric Clinics of North America,* 4:89.

Carter, C.O. 1967. Risks to offspring of incest. *Lancet* 1:436.

Cassem, E.H. 1988. Depression secondary to medical illness. In *American Psychiatric Press Review of Psychiatry,* Vol. 7. A.J. Frances, and R.E. Hales, eds. Washington, D.C.: American Psychiatric Press.

Cavallin, H. 1973. Incest. *Sexual Behavior* 3:19.

Chagnon, N.A. 1974. *Studying the Yänomämo.* New York: Holt, Rinehart and Winston.

———. 1977. *Yänomämo: The Fierce People,* 2nd Edition. New York: Holt, Rinehart and Winston.

———. 1979a. Is reproductive success equal in egalitarian societies? In *Evolutionary Biology and Human Social Behavior: An Anthropological Perspective.* N.A. Chagnon, and W. Irons, editors. North Scituate, MA: Duxbury Press.

———. 1979b. Mate competition, favoring close kin, and village fissioning among the Yänomämo indians. In *Evolutionary Biology and Human Social Behavior: An Anthropological Perspective.* N.A. Chagnon, and W. Irons, editors. North Scituate, MA: Duxbury Press.

———. 1980. Kin-selection theory, kinship, marriage and fitness among the Yänomämo indians. In *Sociobiology: Beyond Nature/Nurture?* G.W. Barlow, and J. Silverberg, editors. Washington, D.C.: American Association for the Advancement of Science.

———. 1982. Nepotism in tribal populations. In *Current Problems in Sociobiology.* King's College Sociobiology Group, editors. Cambridge: Cambridge University Press.

Chagnon, N.A., and Bugos, P.E. 1979. Kin selection and conflict: An analysis of a Yänomämo ax fight. In *Evolutionary Biology and Human Social Behavior: An Anthropological Perspective.* N.A. Chagnon, And W. Irons, editors. North Scituate, MA: Duxbury Press.

Chagnon, N.A. Flinn, M.V., and Melancon, T.F. 1979. Sex-ratio variation among the Yänomämo indians. In *Evolutionary Biology and Human Social Behavior: An Anthropological Perspective.* N.A. Chagnon, and W. Irons, editors. North Scituate, MA: Duxbury Press.

Chagnon, N.A., and Irons, W., eds. 1979. *Evolutionary Biology and Human Social Behavior: An Anthropological Perspective.* North Scituate, MA: Duxbury Press.

Chance, M.R.A. 1962. Social behaviour and primate evolution. In *Culture and the Evolution of Man.* A. Montagu, editor. New York: Oxford University Press.

Charney, D.S., and Heninger, G.R. 1986. Alpha-2 adrenergic and opiate receptor blockade: Synergistic effects on anxiety in healthy subjects. *Archives of General Psychiatry* 43:1037.

Charney, D.S., Nelson, C.J., and Quinlan, D.M. 1981. Personality traits and disorder in depression. *American Journal of Psychiatry* 138:1601.

Chepko-Sade, B.D. 1979. Monkey group splits up. *New Scientist* 82:348.

Chisholm, J.S. 1988. Toward a developmental evolutionary ecology of humans. In *Sociobiological Perspectives on Human Development*. K. MacDonald, ed. New York: Springer-Verlag.

Chodoff, P. 1972. The depressive personality: A critical review. *Archives of General Psychiatry* 27:666.

———. 1982. Hysteria and women. *American Journal of Psychiatry* 139:545.

Chomsky, N. 1975. *Reflections on Language*. New York: Random House.

———. 1980. Rules and representations. *Behavioral and Brain Sciences* 3:1.

Christenson, R., and Blazer, D. 1984. Epidemiology of persecutory ideation in an elderly population in the community. *American Journal of Psychiatry* 141:1088.

Clark, J.T., Smith, E.R., and Davidson, J.M. 1984. Enhancement of sexual motivation in male rats by yohimbine. *Science* 225:847.

Clarkin, J.F., Widiger, T.A., Frances, A., et al. 1983. Prototypic typology and the borderline personality disorder. *Journal of Abnormal Psychology* 92:263.

Clayton, P.J. 1981. The epidemiology of bipolar affective disorder. *Comprehensive Psychiatry* 22:31.

Clutton-Brock, T.H., and Harvey, P.H. 1976. Evolutionary rules and primate societies. In *Growing Points in Ethology*. P.P.G. Bateson, and R.A. Hinde, editors. New York: Cambridge University Press.

Coe, C.L., and Levine, S. 1981. Normal responses to mother-infant separation in nonhuman primates. In *Anxiety: New Research and Changing Concepts*. D. Klein, and J. Rabkin, editors. New York: Raven.

Cohen, M.B., Blake, G., Cohen, R.A., et al. 1954. An intensive study of twelve cases of manic-depressive psychosis. *Psychiatry* 17:103.

Cohen, R. 1961. Marriage instability among the Kanuri of northern Nigeria. *American Anthropologist* 63:1231.

Cole, M., Hood, L., and McDermott, R. 1982. Ecological niche picking. In *Memory Observed: Remembering in Natural Contexts*. U. Neisser, ed. San Francisco: W.H. Freeman.

Conner, R.L., Levine, S., Wertheim, G.A., et al. 1969. Hormonal determinants of aggressive behavior. *Annals of the New York Academy of Science* 159:760.

Cooper, W.S. 1987. Decision theory as a branch of evolutionary theory: A biological derivation of the Savage axioms. *Psychological Review* 94:395.

Coryell, W. 1981. Obsessive-compulsive disorder and primary unipolar depression: Comparisons of background, family history, course, and mortality. *Journal of Nervous and Mental Disorder* 169:220.

Coryell, W., Endicott, J., Reich, T., et al. 1984. A family study of bipolar II disorder. *British Journal of Psychiatry* 145:49.

Coryell, W., and Norten, S.G. 1981. Briquet's syndrome (somatization disorder) and primary depression: Comparison of background and outcome. *Comprehensive Psychiatry* 22:249.

Cosmides, L. 1989. The logic of social exchange: Has natural selection shaped how humans reason? Studies with the Wason selection task. *Cognition* 31:187.

Cosmides, L., and Tooby, J. 1987. From evolution to behavior: Evolutionary psychology as the missing link. In *The Latest on the Best: Essays on Evolution and Optimality*. J. Dupre, ed. Cambridge, MA: MIT Press.

———. 1989. Evolutionary psychology and the generation of culture, part II. Case study: A computational theory of social exchange. *Ethology and Sociobiology* 10:51.

Costello, C.G. 1978. A critical review of Seligman's laboratory experiments on learned helplessness and depression in humans. *Journal of Abnormal Psychology* 87:21.

Cox, F.M., and Campbell, D. 1968. Young children in a new situation with and without their mothers. *Child Development* 39:123.

Crawford, C. 1987. Sociobiology: Of what value to psychology? In *Sociobiology and Psychology: Ideas, Issues, and Applications*. C. Crawford, M. Smith, and D. Krebs, eds. Hillsdale, NJ: Lawrence Erlbaum.

Creese, I., Burt, D.R., and Snyder, S.H. 1976. Dopamine receptor binding predicts clinical and pharmacologic potencies of antischizophrenic drugs. *Science* 192: 481.

Crockenberg, S.B. 1981. Infant irritability, mother responsiveness, and social support influences on the security of mother-infant attachment. *Child Development* 52:857.

Crook, T., and Eliot, J. 1980. Parental death during childhood and adult depression: A critical review of the literature. *Psychological Bulletin* 87:252.

Crutchfield, R.A. 1955. Conformity and character. *American Psychologist* 10:191.

Cutting, J., and Murphy, D. 1988. Schizophrenic thought disorder: A psychological and organic interpretation. *British Journal of Psychiatry* 152:310.

Daly, M., and Wilson, M. 1979. Sex and strategy. *New Scientist* 81:15.

———. 1980. Discriminative parental solicitude: A biological perspective. *Journal of Marriage and the Family* 42:277.

———. 1981. Child maltreatment from a sociobiological perspective. *New Directions for Child Development* 11:93.

———. 1982. Who are newborn babies said to resemble? *Ethology and Sociobiology* 3:69.

———. 1987. Evolutionary psychology and family violence. In *Sociobiology and Psychology: Ideas, Issues and Applications*. C. Crawford, M. Smith, and D. Krebs, eds. Hillsdale, NJ: Lawrence Erlbaum.

Darwin, C. 1859. *The Origin of Species by Means of Natural Selection, or, the Preservation of Favored Races in the Struggle for Life*. London: John Murray.

———. 1871. *The Descent of Man, and Selection in Relation to Sex*. London: John Murray.

Davidson, M., Losonczy, M.F., and Davis, K.L. 1986. Biological hypotheses of schizophrenia. In *American Handbook of Psychiatry*, 2nd Edition, Vol. 8.

Biological Psychiatry. P.A. Berger, and H.K.H. Brodie, editors. New York: Basic Books.

Davies, N.B. 1982. Behaviour and competition for scarce resources. In *Current Problems in Sociobiology.* King's College Sociobiology Group, editors. Cambridge: Cambridge University Press.

Davis, J.M., and Sharma, R.P. 1986. Biological treatment of affective disorders. In *American Handbook of Psychiatry,* 2nd Edition, Vol. 8. *Biological Psychiatry.* P.A. Berger, and H.K.H. Brodie, editors. New York: Basic Books.

Davis, K., and Blake, J. 1956. Social structure and fertility. *Economic Development and Culture Change* 4:211.

Davis, M., and Wallbridge, D. 1981. *Boundary and Space: An Introduction to the Work of D.W. Winnicott.* New York: Brunner/Mazel.

Davis, M.D. 1983. *Game Theory: A Nontechnical Introduction,* revised edition. New York: Basic Books.

DeCasper, A.J., and Fifer, W.P. 1980. Of human bonding: Newborns prefer their mothers' voices. *Science* 208:1174.

DeChateau, P. 1983. Left-sided preferences for holding and carrying newborn infants: Parental holding and carrying during the first week of life. *Journal of Nervous and Mental Disease* 171:241.

DeChateau, P., and Wiberg, B. 1977a. Long-term effect on mother-infant behaviour of extra contact during the first hour post-partum. I. First observations at 36 hours. *Acta Paediatrica Scandinavica* 66:137.

———. 1977b. Long-term effect on mother-infant behaviour of extra contact during the first hour post-partum. II. A follow-up at three months. *Acta Paediatrica Scandinavia* 66:145.

Decina, P., Kestenbaum, C.J., Farber, S., et al. 1983. Clinical and psychological assessment of children of bipolar probands. *American Journal of Psychiatry* 140:548.

DeLozier, P.P. 1982. Attachment theory and child abuse. In *The Place of Attachment in Human Behavior.* C.M. Parkes, and J. Stevenson-Hinde, editors. New York: Basic Books.

Deltito, J.A., Perugi, G., Maremmani, I., et al. 1986. The importance of separation anxiety in the differentiation of panic disorder from agoraphobia. *Psychiatric Developments* 4:227.

Dewsbury, D.A. 1982. Avoidance of incestuous breeding in two species of *Peromyscus* mice. *Biology of Behaviour* 7:157.

Dickemann, M. 1979. Female infanticide, reproductive strategies, and social stratification: A preliminary model. In *Evolutionary Biology and Human Social Behavior: An Anthropological Perspective.* N.A. Chagnon, and W. Irons, editors. North Scituate: MA: Duxbury Press.

Dijkstra, B. 1986. *Idols of Perversity: Fantasies of Feminine Evil in Fin-de-Siecle Culture.* New York: Oxford University Press.

Divale, W.T., and Harris, M. 1976. Population, warfare, and the male supremacist complex. *American Anthropologist* 78:521.

Doane, J.A., West, K.L., Goldstein, M.J., et al. 1981. Parental communication deviance and affective style. *Archives of General Psychiatry* 38:679.

Dobzhansky, T. 1951. *Genetics and the Origin of Species,* 3rd Edition. New York: Columbia University Press.

Docherty, J.P., Fiester, S.J., and Shea, T. 1986. Syndrome diagnosis and personality disorder. In *American Psychiatric Association Annual Review,* Vol. 5. A.J. Frances, and R.E. Hales, editors. Washington, D.C.: American Psychiatric Press.

Dohrenwend, B.P., and Dohrenwend, B.S. 1974. Psychiatric disorders in urban settings. In *American Handbook of Psychiatry,* 2nd Edition, Vol. II. S. Arieti, editor. New York: Basic Books.

Donovan, W.L., Leavitt, L.A., and Balling, J.D. 1978. Maternal physiological responses to infant signals. *Psychophysiology* 15:68.

Dorner, G. 1976. *Hormones and Brain Differentiation.* Amsterdam: Elsevier.

Dorner, G. 1980. Sexual differentiation of the brain. *Vitamins and Hormones* 38:325.

Draper, P., and Harpending, H. 1982. Father absence and reproductive strategy: An evolutionary perspective. *Journal of Anthropological Research* 38:255.

———. 1988. A sociobiological perspective on the development of human reproductive strategies. In *Sociobiological Perspectives on Human Development.* K.B. MacDonald, ed. New York: Springer-Verlag.

Drinka, G.F. 1984. *The Birth of Neurosis: Myth, Malady, and the Victorians.* New York: Simon and Schuster.

Dunham, H.W. 1976. Society, culture, and mental disorder. *Archives of General Psychiatry* 33:147.

Durham, W.H. 1976. Resource competition and human aggression, Part I: A review of primative war. *Quarterly Review of Biology* 51:385.

———. 1978. Toward a coevolutionary theory of human biology and culture. In *The Sociobiology Debate.* A.L. Caplan, editor. New York: Harper and Row.

Durkheim, E. 1950 . *The Rules of Sociological Method.* Glencoe, Ill.: Free Press.

———. 1965. *The Elementary Forms of the Religious Life.* New York: Free Press.

Dweck, C.S., and Leggett, E.L. 1988. A social-cognitive approach to motivation and personality. *Psychological Review* 95:256.

Eagle, M.N. 1984. *Recent Developments in Psychoanalysis: A Critical Evaluation.* New York: McGraw-Hill.

Egeland, B. 1983. Comments on Kopp, Krakow, and Vaughn's chapter. *Minnesota Symposium in Child Psychology* 16:129.

Ehrhardt, A.A., and Meyer-Bahlburg, H.F.L. 1981. Effects of prenatal sex hormones on gender-related behavior. *Science* 211:1312.

Eibl-Eibesfeldt, I. 1970. *Ethology: The Biology of Behaviour.* New York: Holt, Rinehart and Winston.

———. 1973. The expressive behaviour of the deaf-and-blind born. In *Social Communication and Movement.* M. von Cranach, and I. Vine, editors. New York: Academic Press.

Eichelman, B. 1986. The biology and somatic experimental treatment of aggressive disorders. In *American Handbook of Psychiatry,* 2nd Edition, Vol. 8. P.A. Berger and H.K.H. Brodie, editors. New York: Basic Books.

Eimas, P.D. 1985. The perception of speech in early infancy. *Scientific American* 252:46.

Eimas, P.D., Siqueland, E.R., Jusczyk, P. et al. 1971. Speech perception in infants. *Science* 171:303.

Eitinger, L. 1960. The symptomatology of mental disease among refugees in Norway. *Journal of Mental Science* 106:947.

Ekman, P. 1979. About brows: Emotional and conversational signals. In *Human Ethology: Claims and Limits of a New Discipline.* M. von Cranach, K. Foppa, W. Lepenies, et al., editors. New York: Cambridge University Press.

Ellenberger, H.F. 1970. *The Discovery of the Unconscious: The History and Evolution of Dynamic Psychiatry.* New York: Basic Books.

Ellis, A. 1962. *Reason and Emotion in Psychotherapy.* New York: Lyle Stuart.

Ellis, A., and Grieger, R. 1977. *Handbook of Rational Emotive Therapy.* New York: Springer-Verlag.

Ellyson, S.L., and Dovidio, J.F., eds. 1985. *Power, Dominance, and Nonverbal Behavior.* New York: Springer-Verlag.

Ember, C.R. 1978. Myths about hunter-gatherers. *Ethnology* 17:439.

Emde, R.N., Klingman, D.H., Reich, J.H., et al. 1978. Emotional expression in infancy: I. Initial studies of social signaling and an emergent model. In *The Development of Affect.* M. Lewis, and L. Rosenblum, editors. New York: Plenum.

Emde, R.N. and Sorce, J.E. 1983. The rewards of infancy: Emotional availability and maternal referencing. In *Frontiers of Infant Psychiatry,* Vol. 2. J.D. Call, E. Galenson, and R. Tyson, editors. New York: Basic Books.

Engels, F. 1972. *The Origin of the Family, Private Property and the State.* New York: International Publishers.

Epstein, A.W. 1980. Familial imperative ideas and actions: How encoded? *Biological Psychiatry* 15:489.

Epstein, A.W., and Collie, W.R. 1976. Is there a genetic factor in certain dream types? *Biological Psychiatry* 11:359.

Erdman, G., and Janke, W. 1978. Interaction between physiological and cognitive determinants of emotions: Experimental studies on Schachter's theory of emotions. *Biological Psychology* 6:61.

Erickson, M.F., Sroufe, L.A., and Egeland, B. 1985. The relationship between quality of attachment and behavior problems in preschool in a high-risk sample. *Monographs of the Society for Research in Child Development* 50(1–2): 147.

Erikson, E.H. 1950. *Childhood and Society.* New York: W.W. Norton.

———. 1968. *Identity: Youth and Crisis.* New York: W.W. Norton.

———. 1969. *Gandhi's truth: On the Origin of Militant Nonviolence.* New York: W.W. Norton.

Essock-Vitale, S.M. 1983. The reproductive success of wealthy Americans. *Ethology and Sociobiology* 5:45.

Fabre-Nys, C., Meller, R.E., and Keverne, E.B. 1982. Opiate antagonists stimulate affiliative behaviour in monkeys. *Pharmacology, Biochemistry, and Behavior* 16:653.

Fagan, J.F. 1973. Infants' delayed recognition memory and forgetting. *Journal of Experimental Child Psychology* 16:424.

Fagan, J.F. 1976. Infants' recognition of invariant features of faces. *Child Development* 47:627.

Fairbairn, W.R.D. 1952. *An Object-Relations Theory of the Personality.* New York: Basic Books.

Falcon, S., Ryan, C., Chamberlain, K., et al. 1985. Tricyclics: Possible treatment for posttraumatic stress disorder. *Journal of Clinical Psychiatry* 46:385.

Fantz, R. 1963. Pattern vision in newborn infants. *Science* 140:296.

Faravelli, C., and Pallanti, S. 1989. Recent life events and panic disorder. *American Journal of Psychiatry* 146:622.

Faravelli, C., Webb, T., Ambonetti, A., et al. 1985. Prevalence of traumatic early life events in 31 agoraphobic patients with panic attacks. *American Journal of Psychiatry* 142:1493.

Farber, S.L. 1981. *Identical Twins Reared Apart: A Reanalysis.* New York: Basic Books.

Farris, R.E.L., and Dunham, H.W. 1939. *Mental Disorders in Urban Areas: An Ecological Study of Schizophrenia and Other Psychoses.* Chicago: University of Chicago Press.

Fawcett, J., and Kravitz, H.M. 1983. Anxiety syndromes and their relationship to depressive illness. *Journal of Clinical Psychiatry* 44:8.

Feldman, M.W., Cavelli-Sforza, L.L., and Peck, J.R. 1985. Gene-culture coevolution: Models for the evolution of altruism with cultural transmission. *Proceedings of the National Academy of Sciences of the United States of America* 82: 5814.

Fenichel, O. 1945. *The Psychoanalytic Theory of Neurosis.* New York: W.W. Norton.

Festinger, L. 1986. The social organization of early human groups. In *Changing Conceptions of Crowd Mind and Behavior.* C.F. Graumann, and S. Moscovici, editors. New York: Springer-Verlag.

Field, T.M., Woodson, R., Greenberg, R., et al. 1982. Discrimination and imitation of facial expressions by neonates. *Science* 218:179.

Finger, S. 1975. Child-holding patterns in western art. *Child Development* 46:267.

Finkelstein, P., Wenegrat, B., and Yalom, I. 1982. Large group awareness training. *Annual Review of Psychology* 33:515.

Firth, R. 1957. *We the Tikopia,* 2nd Ed. London: Allen and Unwin.

Fischman, M., Schuster, C.R., and Uhlenhuth, E.H. 1977. Extension of animal models to clinical evaluation of antianxiety agents. In *Animal Models in Psychiatry and Neurology.* I. Hanin, and E. Usdin, eds. New York: Pergamon.

Fisher, R.A. 1930. *The Genetical Theory of Natural Selection.* 2nd Ed. New York: Dover.

Fisher, S., and Greenberg, R.P. 1985. *The Scientific Credibility of Freud's Theories and Therapy.* New York: Columbia University Press.

Fodor, J.A. 1980. Reply to Putnam. In *Language and Learning: The Debate*

Between Jean Piaget and Noam Chomsky. M. Piattelli-Palmarini, ed. Cambridge, MA: Harvard University Press.

————. 1983. *The Modularity of Mind: An Essay on Faculty Psychology.* Cambridge, MA: MIT Press.

Fortes, M. 1949. *The Web of Kinship among the Tallensi.* Oxford: Oxford University Press.

Fox, R. 1967. *Kinship and Marriage: An Anthropological Perspective.* Baltimore: Penguin.

————. 1979. Kinship categories as natural categories. In *Evolutionary Biology and Human Social Behavior: An Anthropological Perspective.* N.A. Chagnon, and W. Irons, editors. North Scituate, MA: Duxbury Press.

————. 1980. *The Red Lamp of Incest.* New York: E.P. Dutton.

Frances, A., Sweeney, J., and Clarkin, J. 1985. Do psychotherapies have specific effects. *American Journal of Psychotherapy* 39:159.

Frances, A.J., and Widiger, T. 1986. The classification of personality disorders: An overview of problems and solutions. In *American Psychiatric Association Annual Review,* Vol. 5. A.J. Frances, and R.E. Hales, editors. Washington, D.C.: American Psychiatric Press.

Frank, J.D. 1974. *Persuasion and Healing,* Rev. Ed. New York: Schocken Books.

Freud, A. 1966. *The Ego and the Mechanisms of Defense.* New York: International Universities Press.

Freud, S. 1901. The psychopathology of everyday life. In *The Standard Edition of the Complete Psychological Works of Sigmund Freud,* Vol. 6. J. Strachey, trans. London: Hogarth Press.

————. 1905. Three essays on the theory of sexuality. In *The Standard Edition of the Complete Psychological Works of Sigmund Freud,* Vol. 7. J. Strachey, trans. London: Hogarth Press.

————. 1907. Obsessive actions and religious practices. In *The Standard Edition of the Complete Psychological Works of Sigmund Freud,* Vol. 9. J. Strachey, trans. London: Hogarth Press.

————. 1911. Psychoanalytic notes upon an autobiographical account of a case of paranoia. In *The Standard Edition of the Complete Psychological Works of Sigmund Freud,* Vol. 12. J. Strachey, trans. London: Hogarth Press.

————. 1913. Totem and taboo. In *The Standard Edition of the Complete Psychological Works of Sigmund Freud,* Vol. 13. J. Strachey, trans. London: Hogarth Press.

————. 1914. On narcissism: An introduction. In *The Standard Edition of the Complete Psychological Works of Sigmund Freud,* Vol. 14. J. Strachey, trans. London: Hogarth Press.

————. 1916. Mourning and melancholia. In *The Standard Edition of the Complete Psychological Works of Sigmund Freud,* Vol. 14. J. Strachey, trans. London: Hogarth Press.

————. 1917. Introductory lectures on psychoanalysis. In *The Standard Edition of the Complete Psychological Works of Sigmund Freud,* Vols. 15 and 16. J. Strachey, trans. London: Hogarth Press.

————. 1919. Preface to Reik's Ritual: Psycho-analytic Studies. In *The Standard*

Edition of the Complete Psychological Works of Sigmund Freud, Vol. 17. J. Strachey, trans. London: Hogarth Press.

———. 1921. Group psychology and the analysis of the ego. In *The Standard Edition of the Complete Psychological Works of Sigmund Freud,* Vol. 18. J. Strachey, trans. London: Hogarth Press.

———. 1923. The ego and the id. In *The Standard Edition of the Complete Psychological Works of Sigmund Freud,* Vol. 19, J. Strachey, trans. London: Hogarth Press.

———. 1927. The future of an illusion. In *The Standard Edition of the Complete Psychological Works of Sigmund Freud,* Vol. 21. J. Strachey, trans. London: Hogarth Press.

———. 1939. Moses and monotheism. In *The Standard Edition of the Complete Psychological Works of Sigmund Freud,* Vol. 23. London: Hogarth Press.

———. 1940. An outline of psychoanalysis. In *The Standard Edition of the Complete Psychological Works of Sigmund Freud,* Vol. 23. J. Strachey, trans. London: Hogarth Press.

Friedlander, B.Z. 1970. Receptive language development in infancy. *Merrill-Palmer Quarterly* 16:7.

Fromm, E. 1961. *Marx's Concept of Man.* New York: Frederick Ungar.

Fuller, J.L. 1987. What can genes do? In *Sociobiology and Psychology: Ideas, Issues and Applications.* C. Crawford, M. Smith, and D. Krebs, eds. Hillsdale, NJ: Lawrence Erlbaum.

Fyer, A.J., and Sandberg, D. 1988. Pharmacologic treatment of panic disorder. In *American Psychiatric Press Review of Psychiatry,* Vol. 7. A.J. Frances, and R.E. Hales, eds. Washington, D.C.: American Psychiatric Press.

Gadgil, M., and Bossert, W.H. 1970. Life historical consequences of natural selection. *American Naturalist* 104:1.

Galanter, M. 1978. The "Relief Act": A sociobiological model for neurotic distress and large-group theory. *American Journal of Psychiatry* 135:588.

———. 1983. Unification Church ("Moonie") dropouts: Psychological readjustment after leaving a charismatic religious group. *American Journal of Psychiatry* 140:984.

———. 1989. *Cults: Faith, Healing, and Coercion.* New York: Oxford University Press.

Garbutt, J.C., Loosen, P.T., Tipermas, A., et al. 1983. The TRE test in patients with borderline personality disorder. *Psychiatry Research* 9:107.

Garcia, J., and Koelling, R.A. 1966. Relation of cue to consequence in avoidance learning. *Psychonomic Science* 4:123.

Garcia, J., McGowan, B.K., and Green, K.F. 1972. Biological constraints on conditioning. In *Classical Conditioning II: Current Research and Theory.* A.H. Black, and W.F. Prokasy, eds. New York: Appleton-Century-Crofts.

Gardner, B.T., and Wallach, L. 1965. Shapes of figures identified as a baby's head. *Perceptual and Motor Skills* 20:135.

Gardner, R., Jr. 1982. Mechanisms in manic-depressive disorder. *Archives of General Psychiatry* 39:1436.

Gedo, J.E. 1979. *Beyond Interpretation.* New York: International Universities Press.

————. 1980. Reflections on some current controversies in psychoanalysis. *Journal of the American Psychoanalytic Association* 28:363.

Geiser, R.L. 1979. *Hidden Victims: The Sexual Abuse of Children.* Boston: Beacon Press.

George, C., and Main, M. 1979. Social interactions of young abused children: Approach, avoidance, and aggression. *Child Development* 50:306.

Gerner, R.H., and Bunney, W.E., Jr. 1986. Biological hypotheses of affective disorders. In *American Handbook of Psychiatry,* 2nd Ed., Volume 8. *Biological Psychiatry.* P.A. Berger, and H.K.H. Brodie, editors. New York: Basic Books.

Gershon, E.S., Baron, M., and Leckman, F. 1975. Genetic models of the transmission of affective disorders. *Journal of Psychiatric Research* 12:301.

Gershon, E.S., Cromer, M., and Klerman, G.L. 1968. Hostility and depression. *Psychiatry* 31:224.

Gershon, E.S., McKnew, D., Cytryn, L., et al. 1985. Diagnoses in school-age children of bipolar affective disorder patients and normal controls. *Journal of Affective Disorders* 8:283.

Geshwind, N. 1979. Specializations of the human brain. *Scientific American* 241:180.

Gessa, G.L., and Tagliomonte, A. 1974. Possible role of brain serotonin and dopamine in controlling male sexual behavior. *Advances in Biochemical Psychopharmacology* 2:217.

Ghiselin, M.T. 1974. *The Economy of Nature and the Evolution of Sex.* Berkeley: University of California Press.

Gilbert, J. 1980. *Interpreting Psychological Test Data,* Vol. 2. New York: Van Nostrand Reinhold.

Gittelman, R., and Klein, D.F. 1973. School phobia: Diagnostic considerations in the light of imipramine effects. *Journal of Nervous and Mental Disease* 156: 199.

————. 1984. Relationship between separation anxiety and panic and agoraphobic disorders. *Psychopathology* 17:suppl. 1, 56.

Glantz, K., and Pearce, J. 1989. *Exiles from Eden: Psychotherapy from an Evolutionary Perspective.* New York: W.W. Norton.

Gluck, J.P., and Sackett, G.P. 1974. Frustration and self-aggression in social-isolate rhesus monkeys. *Journal of Abnormal Psychology* 83:331.

Goldberg, A., Ed. 1978. *The Psychology of the Self: A Casebook.* New York: International Universities Press.

————. 1980. *Advances in Self Psychology.* New York: International Universities Press.

Goldberg, T.E., Weinberger, D.R., Berman, K.F., et al. 1987. Further evidence for dementia of the prefrontal type in schizophrenia?: A controlled study of teaching the Wisconsin Card Sorting Test. *Archives of General Psychiatry* 44:1008.

Goldfoot, D.A. 1977. Sociosexual behaviors of nonhuman primates during development and maturity: Social and hormonal relationships. In *Behavioral Primatology: Advances in Research and Theory,* Vol. 1. A.M. Schrier, ed. Hillsdale, NJ: Lawrence Erlbaum.

Goldin, L.R., and Gershon, E.S. 1988. The genetic epidemiology of major depressive illness. In *American Psychiatric Press Review of Psychiatry,* Vol. 7. A.J. Frances, and R.E. Hales, eds. Washington, D.C.: American Psychiatric Press.

Goodman, A.B., Siegel, C., Craig, T.J., et al. 1983. The relationship between socioeconomic class and prevalence of schizophrenia, alcoholism, and affective disorders treated by inpatient care in a suburban area. *American Journal of Psychiatry* 140:166.

Goodwin, D., and Guze, S. 1984. *Psychiatric Diagnosis,* 3rd Ed. New York: Oxford University Press.

Goodwin, F.K., and Roy-Byrne, P. 1987. Treatment of bipolar disorders. In *American Psychiatric Association Annual Review,* Vol. 6. R.E. Hales, and A.J. Frances, editors. Washington, D.C.: American Psychiatric Press.

Gorman, J.M., Askanazi, J., Liebowitz, M., et al. 1984. Response to hyperventilation in panic disorder. *American Journal of Psychiatry* 141:857.

Gotlib, I.H., Mount, J.H., Cordy, N.I., et al. 1988. Depression and perceptions of early parenting: A longitudinal investigation. *British Journal of Psychiatry* 152:24.

Gottesman, I.I., and Shields, J. 1982. *Schizophrenia: The Epigenetic Puzzle.* Cambridge: Cambridge University Press.

Gouldner, A. 1960. The norm of reciprocity: A preliminary statement. *American Sociological Review* 47:73.

Goy, R.W., and McEwan, B.S. 1980. *Sexual Differentiation in the Brain.* Cambridge, MA: MIT Press.

Gray, J.A., and Drewett, R.F. 1977. The genetics and development of sex differences. In *Handbook of Modern Personality Theory.* R.B. Cattell, and R.M. Dreger, editors. New York: Halsted Press.

Gray, M. 1978. *Neuroses: A Comprehensive and Critical View.* New York: Van Nostrand Reinhold.

Green, M.A., and Curtis, G.C. 1988. Personality disorders in panic patients: Response to termination of antipanic medication. *Journal of Personality Disorders* 2:303.

Greenberg, J.R., and Mitchell, S.A. 1983. *Object Relations in Psychoanalytic Theory.* Cambridge, MA: Harvard University Press.

Greenberg, R.P., and Bornstein, R.F. 1988. The dependent personality: II. Risk for psychological disorders. *Journal of Personality Disorders* 2:136.

Griez, E., and Van den Hout, M.A. 1983. Treatment of photophobia by exposure to CO2 induced anxiety symptoms. *Journal of Nervous and Mental Disease* 175:506.

Grinker, R. 1979. Diagnosis of borderlines: A discussion. *Schizophrenia Bulletin* 5:47.

Grossmann, K., Grossmann, K.E., Spangler, G., et al. 1985. Maternal sensitivity and newborns' orientation responses as related to quality of attachment in northern Germany. *Monographs of the Society for Research in Child Development* 50(1–2):233.

Grosz, H.J., and Farmer, B.B. 1972. Pitts and McClure's lactate-anxiety study revisited. *British Journal of Psychiatry* 120:415.

Grumet, G.W. 1983. Eye contact: The core of interpersonal relatedness. *Psychiatry* 46:172.

Grunhaus, L. 1988. Clinical and psychobiological characteristics of simultaneous panic disorder and major depression. *American Journal of Psychiatry* 145: 1214.

Grunhaus, L., Gloger, S., and Weisstub, E. 1981. Panic attacks: A review of treatments and pathogenesis. *Journal of Nervous and Mental Disease* 169:608.

Gruter, M., and Bohannon, P., eds. 1983. *Law, Biology and Culture: The Evolution of Law.* Santa Barbara, CA: Ross-Erikson.

Guidubaldi, J., Cleminshaw, H.K., Perry, J.D., et al. 1983. The legacy of parental divorce. *School Psychology Review* 12:300.

Gunderson, J.G. 1979. Individual psychotherapy. In *Disorders of the Schizophrenic Spectrum.* L. Bellak, editor. New York: Basic Books.

Gunderson, J.G., Carpenter, W., and Strauss, J. 1975. Borderline and schizophrenic patients: A comparative study. *American Journal of Psychiatry* 132:1257.

Gunderson, J.G., Kerr, J., and Englund, D.W. 1980. The families of borderlines. *Archives of General Psychiatry* 37:27.

Gunderson, J.G., and Kolb, J. 1978. Discriminating features of borderline patients. *American Journal of Psychiatry* 135:792.

Guntrip, H. 1961. *Personality Structure and Human Interaction: The Developing Synthesis of Psychodynamic Theory.* New York: International Universities Press.

———. 1971. *Psychoanalytic Theory, Therapy and the Self.* New York: Basic Books.

Haldane, J.B.S. 1932. *The Causes of Evolution.* London: Longmans and Green.

Hales, D.J., Lozoff, B., Sosa, R., et al. 1977. Defining the limits of the maternal sensitive period. *Developmental Medicine and Child Neurology* 19:454.

Hall, K.R.L. 1960. Social vigilance behaviour of the chacma baboon, *Papio Ursinus. Behaviour* 16:261.

Hallam, R.S. 1985. *Anxiety: Psychological Perspectives on Panic and Agoraphobia.* New York: Academic Press.

Hamilton, W.D. 1964. The genetical evolution of social behavior. *Journal of Theoretical Biology* 7:1.

———. 1971. Geometry for the selfish herd. *Journal of Theoretical Biology* 31:295.

Hammerstein, P. 1981. The role of asymmetries in animal contents. *Animal Behaviour* 29:193.

Harlow, H.F. 1971. *Learning to Love.* San Francisco: Albion.

Harlow, H.F., and Harlow, M. 1965. The affectional system. In *Behavior of Nonhuman Primates.* A. Schrier, H. Harlow, and F. Stollnitz, editors. New York: Academic Press.

Harlow, H.F., McGaugh, J., and Thompson, R.F. 1971. *Psychology.* San Francisco: Albion.

Harlow, H.F., and Zimmerman, R.R. 1959. Affectional responses in the infant monkey. *Science* 130:421.

Harper, R.G. 1985. Power, dominance and nonverbal behavior: An overview. In *Power, Dominance, and Nonverbal Behavior*. S.L. Ellyson, and J.F. Dovidio, editors. New York: Springer-Verlag.

Harrington, M. 1983. *The Politics of God's Funeral: The Spiritual Crisis of Western Civilization*. New York: Penguin.

Hartmann, E. 1984. *The Nightmare: The Psychology and Biology of Terrifying Dreams*. New York: Basic Books.

Hartmann, E., Russ, D., van der Kolk, B., et al. 1981. A preliminary study of the personality of the nightmare sufferer: Relationship to schizophrenia and creativity? *American Journal of Psychiatry* 138:794.

Hartmann, H. 1952. The mutual influence in the development of ego and id. *Psychoanalytic Study of the Child* 7:9.

———. 1953. Contribution to the metapsychology of schizophrenia. *Psychoanalytic Study of the Child* 8:177.

Harvey, N.S. 1988. Serial cognitive profiles in levodopa-induced hypersexuality. *British Journal of Psychiatry* 153:833.

Hathout, H.M. 1963. Some aspects of female circumcision. *Journal of Obstetrics and Gynecology of the British Commonwealth* 70:505.

Havens, L. 1987. *Approaches to the Mind: Movement of the Psychiatric Schools from Sects toward Science*. Cambridge, MA: Harvard University Press.

Hecaen, H., and Albert, M.L. 1975. Disorders of mental functioning related to frontal lobe pathology. In *Psychiatric Aspects of Neurologic Disease*. D.F. Benson, and D. Blumer, editors. New York: Grune and Stratton.

Herbert, J. 1976. Hormonal basis of sex differences in rats, monkeys, and humans. *New Scientist* 70:284.

Herbert, M.E., and Jacobson, S. 1967. Late paraphrenia. *British Journal of Psychiatry* 113:461.

Herman, J.L. 1986. Histories of violence in an outpatient population. *American Journal of Orthopsychiatry* 56:137.

Herman, J.L., Perry, J.C., and van der Kolk, B.A. 1989. Childhood trauma in borderline personality disorder. *American Journal of Psychiatry* 146:490.

Herold, E.S., and Goodwin, M.S. 1981. Adamant virgins, potential nonvirgins, and nonvirgins. *Journal of Sex Research* 17:97.

Heston, L., and Denny, D. 1969. Interactions between early life experiences and biological features in schizophrenia. In *Transmissions of Schizophrenia*. D. Rosenthal, and S.S. Kety, editors. Oxford: Pergamon Press.

Hetherington, E.M. 1972. Effects of father absence on personality development in adolescent daughters. *Developmental Psychology* 7:313.

———. 1979. Divorce: A child's perspective. *American Psychologist* 34:851.

Hill, J.L. 1974. *Peromyscus*: Effect of early pairing on reproduction. *Science* 186:1042.

Hinde, R.A., and Spencer-Booth, Y. 1967. The behaviour of socially living rhesus monkeys in their first two and a half years. *Animal Behaviour* 15:169.

———. 1971. Effects of brief separation from mother on rhesus monkeys. *Science* 173:111.

Hinde, R.A., and Stevenson-Hinde, J. 1973. *Constraints on Learning*. London: Academic Press.

————. 1976. Towards understanding relationships: Dynamic stability. In *Growing Points in Ethology.* P.P.G. Bateson, and R.A. Hinde, editors. New York: Cambridge University Press.

Hinsie, L.E., and Campbell, R.J. 1970. *Psychiatric Dictionary,* 4th edition. New York: Oxford University Press.

Hippler, A.E. 1974. *Hunter's Point: A Black Ghetto.* New York: Basic Books.

Hirschfield, R.M.A. 1986. Personality disorders: Foreword. In *American Psychiatric Association Annual Review,* Vol. 5. A.J. Frances, and R.E. Hales, editors. Washington, D.C.: American Psychiatric Press.

Hirschfield, R.M.A., Klerman, G.L., Clayton, P.J., et al. 1983. Personality and depression: Empirical findings. *Archives of General Psychiatry* 40:993.

Hodges, W.F., and Bloom, B.L. 1984. Parents' reports of children's adjustment to marital separation: A longitudinal study. *Journal of Divorce* 8:33.

Hodges, W.F., Buchsbaum, H.K., and Tierney, C.W. 1983. Parent-child relasionships and adjustment in preschool children in divorced and intact families. *Journal of Divorce* 7:43.

Hoffman, M. 1982. Development of prosocial motivation: Empathy and guilt. In *The Development of Prosocial Behavior.* N. Eisenberg, ed. New York: Academic Press.

Hogben, G.L., and Cornfield, R.B. 1981. Treatment of traumatic war neurosis with phenelzine. *Archives of General Psychiatry* 38:440.

Holmes, W.G., and Sherman, P.W. 1983. Kin recognition in animals. *American Scientist* 71:46.

Hood, R.W. 1978. The usefulness of the indiscriminately pro and anti categories of religious orientation. *Journal for the Scientific Study of Religion* 17:419.

Hoogland, J.L. 1982. Prairie dogs avoid extreme inbreeding. *Science* 215:1639.

Hornstein, H.A. 1978. Promotive tension and prosocial behavior: A Lewinian analysis. In *Altruism, Sympathy, and Helping: Psychological and Sociological Principles.* L. Wispe, ed. New York: Academic Press.

Horowitz, M.J., Wilner, N., Kaltreider, N., et al. 1980. Signs and symptoms of posttraumatic stress disorder. *Archives of General Psychiatry* 37:85.

Howard, J.L., and Pollard, G.T. 1977. The Geller Conflict Test: A model of anxiety and a screening procedure for anxiolytics. In *Animal Models in Psychiatry and Neurology.* I. Hanin, and E. Usdin, eds. New York: Pergamon Press.

Hrdina, P.D., Kulmiz, P. von, and Stretch, R. 1979. Pharmacologic modification of experimental depression in infant macaques. *Psychopharmacology* 64:89.

Hrdy, S.B. 1974. Male-male competition and infanticide among the langurs (*Presbytis entellus*) of Abu' Rajasthan. *Folia Primatologica* 22:19.

————. 1977. Infanticide as a primate reproductive strategy. *American Scientist* 65:40.

————. 1981. *The Woman that Never Evolved.* Cambridge: Harvard University Press.

Hudson, J.I., Laffer, P.S., and Pope, H.G. 1982. Bulimia related to affective disorders by family history and response to dexamethasone suppression test. *American Journal of Psychiatry* 139:685.

Hudson, J.I., Pope, H.G., Jonas, J.M., et al. 1983. Phenomenologic relationship of eating disorders to major affective disorder. *Psychiatry Research* 9:345.

Humphrey, N.K. 1976. The social function of intellect. In *Growing Points in Ethology.* P.P.G. Bateson, and R.A. Hinde, editors. New York: Cambridge University Press.

Hunt, R.A., and King, M.B. 1971. The intrinsic-extrinsic concept: A review and evaluation. *Journal for the Scientific Study of Religion* 10:339.

Ingold, T. 1986. *Evolution and Social Life.* London: Cambridge University Press.

Insel, T., and Murphy, D.L. 1981. The psychopharmacological treatment of obsessive compulsive disorder: A review. *Journal of Clinical Psychopharmacology* 1:304.

Irons, W. 1979. Investment and primary social dyads. In *Evolutionary Biology and Human Social Behavior: An Anthropological Perspective.* N.A. Chagnon, and W. Irons, editors. North Scituate, MA: Duxbury Press.

———. 1980. Is Yomut social behavior adaptive? In *Sociobiology: Beyond Nature/Nurture? Reports, Definitions and Debate.* G.W. Barlow, and J. Silverberg, editors. Washington, D.C.: American Association for the Advancement of Science.

———. 1983. Human female reproductive strategies. In *Social Behavior of Female Vertebrates.* S.K. Wasser, editor. New York: Academic Press.

Itani, J., and Nishimura, A. 1973. The study of infrahuman culture in Japan: A review. In *Precultural Primate Behavior.* E.W. Menzel, editor. Basel, Switzerland: Karger.

Itani, J., and Suzuki, A. 1967. The social unit of chimpanzees. *Primates* 8:355.

Itoigawa, N., Negayama, K., and Kondo, K. 1981. Experimental study on sexual behavior between mother and son in Japanese monkeys (*Macaca Fuscata*). *Primates* 22:494.

Izard, C.E. 1978. On the ontogenesis of emotions and emotion-cognition relationship in infancy. In *The Development of Affect.* M. Lewis, and L.A. Rosenblum, editors. New York: Plenum Press.

Jacobs, R.C., and Campbell, D.T. 1961. The perpetuation of an arbitrary tradition through several generations of a laboratory microculture. *Journal of Abnormal and Social Psychology* 62:649.

Jacobson, R. 1986. Disorders of facial recognition, social behaviour and affect after combined bilateral amygdalotomy and subcaudate tractotomy: A clinical and experimental study. *Psychological Medicine* 16:439.

Jakimow-Venulet, B. 1981. Hereditary factors in the pathogenesis of affective illness. *British Journal of Psychiatry* 139:450.

James, W. 1890. *The Principles of Psychology.* New York: Henry Holt.

Jaspers, K. 1963. *General Psychopathology.* Chicago: University of Chicago Press.

Jenner, F.A. 1978. Psychiatry, biology and morals. In *Morality as a Biological Phenomenon.* G.S. Stent, editor. Berlin: Dahlem Konferenzen.

Jenni, D.A., and Jenni, M.A. 1976. Carrying behavior in humans: Analysis of sex differences. *Science* 194:859.

Joffe, R.T., Swinson, R.P., and Regan, J.J. 1988. Personality features of obsessive-compulsive disorder. *American Journal of Psychiatry* 145:1127.

Johansen, K.H. 1983. Transitional experience of a borderline patient. *Journal of Nervous and Mental Disease* 171:126.

Jung, C.G. 1919. Instinct and the unconscious. In *The Collected Works of Carl G.*

Jung, Vol. 8. R.F.C. Hull, translator. Princeton, NJ: Princeton University Press.

Justice, B., and Justice, R. 1979. *The Broken Taboo.* New York: Human Sciences Press.

Kaplan, H.I., and Sadock, B.J., eds. 1985. *Comprehensive Textbook of Psychiatry,* 4th Edition. Baltimore: Williams and Wilkins.

Karlson, J. 1966. *The Biological Basis for Schizophrenia.* Springfield: Charles C. Thomas.

Kass, F., Skodol, A.E., Charles, E., et al. 1985. Scaled ratings of DSM-III personality disorders. *American Journal of Psychiatry* 142:627.

Kauffman, C., Grunebaum, H., Cohler, B., et al. 1979. Superkids: Competent children of psychotic mothers. *American Journal of Psychiatry* 136:1398.

Kaufman, I.C., and Rosenblum, L.A. 1967. Depression in infant monkeys separated from their mothers. *Science* 155:1030.

Kawai, M. 1965. New acquired pre-cultural behavior of the natural troop of Japanese monkeys on Koshima Islet. *Primates* 6:1.

Kay, D.W.K., and Roth, M. 1961. Environmental and hereditary factors in the schizophrenias of old age ("late paraphrenia") and their bearing on the general problems of causation in schizophrenia. *Journal of Mental Science* 107:649.

Keating, C.F. 1985. Human dominance signals: The primate in us. In *Power, Dominance, and Nonverbal Behavior.* S.L. Ellyson, and J.F. Dovidio, editors. New York: Springer-Verlag.

Keller, M.B. 1988. Diagnostic issues and clinical course of unipolar illness. In *American Psychiatric Press Review of Psychiatry,* Vol. 7. A.J. Frances, and R.E. Holmes, eds. Washington, D.C.: American Psychiatric Press.

Kellerman, H. 1980. A structural model of emotion and personality: Psychoanalytic and sociobiological implications. In *Emotion: Theory, Research, and Experience.* Vol. I: *Theories of Emotion.* R. Plutchik, and H. Kellerman, eds. New York: Academic Press.

Kelly, D., Mitchell-Heggs, N., and Sherman, D. 1971. Anxiety and lactate effects assessed clinically and physiologically. *British Journal of Psychiatry* 119:129.

Kendler, K.S. 1982. Demography of paranoid psychosis (delusional disorder). *Archives of General Psychiatry* 39:890.

Kendler, K.S., Gruenberg, A., and Strauss, J. 1981a. An independent analysis of the Copenhagen sample of the Danish adoption study of schizophrenia, II: The relationship between schizotypal personality disorder and schizophrenia. *Archives of General Psychiatry* 38:982.

Kendler, K.S., Gruenberg, A., and Strauss, J. 1981b. An independent analysis of the Copenhagen sample of the Danish adoption study of schizophrenia, III: The relationship between paranoid psychosis (delusional disorder) and the schizophrenia spectrum disorders. *Archives of General Psychiatry* 38:985.

Kendler, K.S., and Hays, P. 1981. Paranoid psychosis (delusional disorder) and schizophenia: A family history study. *Archives of General Psychiatry* 38:547.

Kendler, K.S., Masterson, C.C., and Davis, K.L. 1985. Psychiatric illness in first-degree relatives of patients with paranoid psychosis, schizophrenia and medical illness. *British Journal of Psychiatry* 147:524.

Kendler, K.S., Masterson, C.C., Ungaro, R., et al. 1984. A family history study of schizophrenia related personality disorders. *American Journal of Psychiatry* 141:424.

Kernberg, O.F. 1975. *Borderline Conditions and Pathological Narcissism.* New York: Jason Aronson.

Kety, S.S. 1983. Mental illness in the biological and adoptive relatives of schizophrenic adoptees: Findings relevant to genetic and environmental factors in etiology. *American Journal of Psychiatry* 140:720.

Kinsey, A.C., Pomeroy, W.B., and Martin, C.E. 1948. *Sexual Behavior in the Human Male.* Philadelphia: W.B. Saunders.

Kinsey, A.C., Pomeroy, W.B., Martin, C.E., et al. 1953. *Sexual Behavior in the Human Female.* Philadelphia: W.B. Saunders.

Klaus, M.H., Jerauld, R., Kreger, N.C., et al. 1972. Maternal attachment: Importance of the first post-partum days. *New England Journal of Medicine* 286:460.

Klein, D. 1964. Delineation of two drug-responsive anxiety syndromes. *Psychopharmacologia* 5:397.

———. 1975. Psychopharmacology and the borderline patient. In *Borderline States in Psychiatry.* J.E. Mack, ed. New York: Grune and Stratton.

———. 1980. Anxiety reconceptualized: Early experience with imipramine and anxiety. *Comprehensive Psychiatry* 21:411.

Klein, S.D. 1980. Class, culture, and health. In *Maxcy-Rosenau Public Health and Preventive Medicine,* 11th edition. M.J. Rosenau, ed. New York: Appleton-Century-Croft.

Klerman, G.L., Weissman, M.M., Rounsaville, B.J. et al. 1984. *Interpersonal Psychotherapy of Depression.* New York: Basic Books

Kline, P. 1972. *Fact and Fantasy in Freudian Theory.* London: Methuen.

Kling, A. 1972. Effects of amygdalectomy on social-affective behavior in non-human primates. In *Neurobiology of the Amygdala.* B.E. Eleftherion, editor. New York: Plenum Press.

———. 1986. The anatomy of aggression and affiliation. In *Emotion: Theory, Research, and Experience,* Vol. 3. *Biological Foundations of Emotion.* R. Plutchick, and H. Kellerman, editors. New York: Academic Press.

Kling, A., and Steklis, H.D. 1976. A neural substrate for affiliative behavior in nonhuman primates. *Brain and Behavioral Evolution* 13:216.

Knoedel, J. 1977. Breast feeding and population growth. *Science* 198:1111.

Koenigsberg, H., Kernberg, O., Schomer, J. 1983. Diagnosing borderline conditions in an outpatient setting. *Archives of General Psychiatry* 40:49.

Kohut, H. 1971. *The Analysis of the Self.* New York: International Universities Press.

———. 1972. Thoughts on narcissism and narcissistic rage. *The Psychoanalytic Study of the Child* 27:360.

———. 1977. *The Restoration of the Self.* New York: International Universities Press.

————. 1979. The two analyses of Mr. Z. *International Journal of Psycho-Analysis* 60:3.

————. 1984. *How Does Analysis Cure?* A. Goldberg, and P.E. Stepansky, editors. Chicago: University of Chicago Press.

Kohut, H., and Wolf, E.S. 1978. The disorders of the self and their treatment: An outline. *International Journal of Psycho-Analysis* 59:413.

Konner, M. 1982. *The Tangled Wing: Biological Constraints on the Human Spirit.* New York: Harper and Row.

Kraemer, G.W., and McKinney, W. 1979. Interactions of pharmacological agents altering biogenic amine metabolism and depression. *Journal of Affective Disorders* 1:33.

Kraepelin, E. 1921. *Manic-Depressive Insanity and Paranoia.* Edinburgh: Livingston.

Kramlinger, K.G., Swanson, D.W., and Maruta, T. 1983. Are patients with chronic pain depressed? *American Journal of Psychiatry* 140:747.

Krause, R., Steimer, E., Sanger-Alt, C., et al. 1989. Facial expression of schizophrenic patients and their interaction partners. *Psychiatry* 52:1.

Krebs, D. 1987. The challenge of altruism in biology and psychology. In *Sociobiology and Psychology: Ideas, Issues and Applications.* C. Crawford, M. Smith, and D. Krebs, eds. Hillsdale, NJ: Lawrence Erlbaum.

Krebs, D., Denton, K., and Higgins, N.C. 1988. On the evolution of self-knowledge and self-deception. In *Sociobiological Perspectives on Human Development.* K.B. MacDonald, ed. New York: Springer-Verlag.

Kroll, J., Sines, L., Martin, K., et al. 1983. Borderline personality disorder. Construct validity of the concept. *Archives of General Psychiatry* 38:1021.

Kuhn, R. 1958. The attempted murder of a prostitute. In *Existence.* R. May, E. Angel, and H.F. Ellenberger, editors. New York: Simon and Schuster.

Kummer, H. 1968. *Social Organization of the Hamadryas Baboons: A Field Study.* Chicago: University of Chicago Press.

————. 1978. Analogs of morality among nonhuman primates. In *Morality as a Biological Phenomenon.* G.S. Stent, editor. Berlin: Dahlem Konferenzen.

————. 1979. On the value of social relationships to nonhuman primates: A heuristic scheme. *In Human Ethology: Claims and Limits of a New Discipline.* M. von Cranach, K. Foppa, W. Lepenies, et al., editors. New York: Cambridge University Press.

Kummer, H., Gotz, W., and Angst, W. 1974. Triadic differentiation: An inhibitory process protecting pair bonds in baboons. *Behaviour* 49:62.

Kunz, P.R., Brinkerhoff, M.B., and Hundley, V. 1973. Relationship of income and childlessness. *Social Biology* 20:139.

Kurland, J.A. 1979. Paternity, mother's brother, and human sociality. In *Evolutionary Biology and Human Social Behavior: An Anthropological Perspective.* N.A. Chagnon, and W. Irons, editors. North Scituate, MA: Duxbury Press.

Lack, D. 1954. *The Natural Regulation of Animals.* New York: Oxford University Press.

————. 1966. *Population Studies of Birds.* New York: Oxford University Press.

————. 1968. *Ecological Adaptation for Breeding in Birds.* London: Methuen.

Lambert, W.W., Triandis, L.M., and Wolf, M. 1959. Some correlates of belief in the malevolence and benevolence of supernatural beings: A cross-cultural study. *Journal of Abnormal and Social Psychology* 58:162.

Langton, J. 1979. Darwinism and the behavioral theory of sociocultural evolution: An analysis. *American Journal of Sociology* 85:288.

Larsen, L., and Knapp, R.H. 1964. Sex differences in symbolic conceptions of the deity. *Journal of Projective Techniques* 28:303.

Last, C.G., Barlow, D.H., and O'Brien, G.T. 1984. Precipitants of agoraphobia: Role of stressful life events. *Psychological Reports* 54:567.

Lawick-Goodall, J. van. 1968. The behaviour of free-living chimpanzees in the Gombe Stream Reserve. *Animal Behaviour Monographs* 1:161.

———. 1971. *In the Shadow of Man*. Boston: Houghton Mifflin.

Lazarus, A.A. 1971. *Behavior Therapy and Beyond*. New York: McGraw-Hill.

———. 1974. Multimodal behavioral treatment of depression. *Behavior Therapy* 5:549.

Lazarus, A.A., and Serber, M. 1968. Is systematic desensitization being misapplied? *Psychological Reports* 23:215.

Leacock, E. 1972. Introduction to *The Origin of the Family, Private Property and the State*. F. Engels. New York: International Publishers.

———. 1978. Women's status in egalitarian society: Implications for social evolution. *Current Anthropology* 19:247.

———. 1980. Social behavior, biology and the double standard. In *Sociobiology: Beyond Nature/Nurture? Reports, Definitions and Debate*. G.W. Barlow, and J. Silverberg, editors. Washington, D.C.: American Association for the Advancement of Science.

Leak, G.K., and Christopher, S.B. 1982. Freudian psychoanalysis and sociobiology: A synthesis. *American Psychologist* 37:313.

LeBoeuf, B.J. 1974. Male-male competition and reproductive success in elephant seals. *American Zoology* 14:163.

Leckman, J.F., Merikangas, K.R., Pauls, D.L., et al. 1983. Anxiety disorders and depression: Contradictions between family study data and DSM-III conventions. *American Journal of Psychiatry* 140:880.

Lehmann, H.E. 1985. Affective disorders: Clinical features. In *Comprehensive Textbook of Psychiatry*, 4th Edition. H.I. Kaplan, and B.J. Sadock, editors. Baltimore: Williams and Wilkins.

Lehmann, H.E., and Cancro, R. 1985. Schizophrenia: Clinical features. In *Comprehensive Textbook of Psychiatry*, 4th Edition. H.I. Kaplan, and B.J. Sadock, editors. Baltimore: Williams and Wilkins.

Lenski, G. 1970. *Human Societies: A Macrolevel Introduction to Sociology*. New York: McGraw-Hill.

Lesser, I.M., Rubin, R.T., Pecknold, J.C., et al. 1988. Secondary depression in panic disorder and agoraphobia. I. Frequency, severity, and response to treatment. *Archives of General Psychiatry* 45:437.

Levine, S. 1982. Comparative and psychobiological perspectives on development. In *Minnesota Symposium on Child Psychology*, Vol. 15. W.A. Collins, editor. Hillsdale, NJ: Erlbaum.

Levi-Strauss, C. 1969. *Elementary Structures of Kinship*. Boston: Beacon Press.

Levy, A.B., Dixon, K.N., and Stern, S.L. 1989. How are depression and bulimia related? *American Journal of Psychiatry* 146:162.

Lewin, B.D. 1932. The analysis and structure of a transient hypomania. *Psychoanalytic Quarterly* 1:43.

Lewinsohn, P.M., and Shaffer, M. 1971. Use of home observations as an integral part of the treatment of depression: Preliminary report and case studies. *Journal of Consulting and Clinical Psychology* 37:87.

Lewis, A.J. 1934. Melancholia. *Journal of Mental Science* 80:277.

Lewis, M., and Goldberg, S. 1969. Perceptual-cognitive development in infancy: A generalized expectancy model as a function of mother-infant interaction. *Merrill-Palmer Quarterly* 15:81.

Lewontin, R.C., Rose, S., and Kamin, L.J. 1984. *Not in Our Genes*. New York: Pantheon.

Liberman, A.M. 1979. An ethological approach to language through the study of speech perception. In *Human Ethology: Claims and Limits of a New Discipline*. M. von Cranach, K. Foppa, W. Lepenies, et al., editors. New York: Cambridge University Press.

Libet, J.M., and Lewinsohn, P.M. 1973. Concept of social skills with special reference to the behavior of depressed persons. *Journal of Consulting and Clinical Psychology* 40:304.

Liebowitz, M.R., Fyer, A.J., Gorman, J.M., et al. 1984. Lactate provocation of panics: I. Clinical and behavioral findings. *Archives of General Psychiatry* 41:764.

Liebowitz, M.R., and Klein, D.F. 1981. Interrelationship of hysteroid dysphoria and borderline personality disorder. *Psychiatric Clinics of North America* 4:67.

Lin, M., and Michener, C. 1971. Evolution of sociality in incest. *Quarterly Review of Biology* 47:131.

Lindemann, E. 1960. Psychosocial factors as stress agents. In *Stress and Psychiatric Disorder*. J. M. Tanner, editor. Oxford: Blackwell.

Linehan, M.M. 1987. Dialectical behavior therapy: A cognitive behavioral approach to parasuicide. *Journal of Personality Disorders* 1:328.

Lishman, W.A. 1987. *Organic Psychiatry: The Psychological Consequences of Cerebral Disorder,* 2nd Edition. Oxford: Blackwell.

Littlefield, C.H., and Rushton, J.P. 1986. When a child dies: The sociobiology of berievement. *Journal of Personality and Social Psychology* 51:797.

Lloyd, C. 1980. Life events and depressive disorder reviewed. *Archives of General Psychiatry* 37:529.

Lockard, J.S. 1980. Speculations on the adaptive significance of self-deception. In *The Evaluation of Human Social Behavior*. J.S. Lockard, ed. New York: Elsevier.

Lockhard, J., Daley, P.C., and Gunderson, V.M. 1979. Maternal and paternal differences in infant carrying: U.S. and African data. *American Naturalist* 113:235.

Lopreato, J. 1984. *Human Nature and Biocultural Evolution*. Boston: Allen and Unwin.

Loranger, A.W., Oldham, J.M., and Tulis, E.H. 1982. Familial transmission of DSM-III borderline personality disorder. *Archives of General Psychiatry* 39:795.

Lorenz, K. 1960. *On Aggression*. New York: Harcourt, Brace and World.

———. 1981. *The Foundations of Ethology: The Principal Ideas and Discoveries in Animal Behavior*. New York: Simon and Schuster.

Luisada, P.V., Peele, R., and Pittard, E.A. 1974. The hysterical personality in men. *American Journal of Psychiatry* 131:518.

Lumsden, C.J. 1985. Color categorization: A possible concordance between genes and culture. *Proceedings of the National Academy of Sciences of the United States of America* 85:5805.

———. 1988. Psychological development: Epigenetic rules and gene-culture coevolution. In *Sociobiological Perspectives on Human Development*. K.B. MacDonald, ed. New York: Springer-Verlag.

———. 1989. Does culture need genes? *Ethology and Sociobiology* 10:11.

Lumsden, C.J., and Wilson, E.O. 1981. *Genes, Mind, and Culture: The Coevolutionary Process*. Cambridge, MA: Harvard University Press.

———. 1983. *Promethean Fire: Reflections on the Origin of Mind*. Cambridge, MA: Harvard University Press.

———. 1985. The relation between biological and cultural evolution. *Journal of Social and Biological Structures* 8:343.

Luria, A.R. 1981. *Language and Cognition*. New York: Wiley.

MacArthur, R.H., and Wilson E.O. 1967. *The Theory of Island Biogeography*. Princeton, NJ: Princeton University Press.

Maccoby, E.E., and Jacklin, C.N. 1974. *The Psychology of Sex Differences*. Palo Alto, CA: Stanford University Press.

MacDonald, K.B. 1988a. The interfaces between sociobiology and developmental psychology. In *Sociobiological Perspectives on Human Development*. K.B. MacDonald, ed. New York: Springer-Verlag.

———. 1988b. Sociobiology and the cognitive-development tradition in moral development research. In *Sociobiological Perspectives on Human Development*. K.B. MacDonald, ed. New York: Springer-Verlag.

———. 1988c. Socialization in the context of the family: A sociobiological perspective. In *Sociobiological Perspectives on Human Development*. K.B. MacDonald, ed. New York: Springer-Verlag.

———. 1989. The plasticity of human social organization and behavior. *Ethology and Sociobiology* 10:171.

MacFarlane, J. 1975. Olfaction in the development of social preferences in the human neonate. In *Parent-Infant Interaction*. M. Hofer, editor. Amsterdam: Elsevier.

Mackey, W.C. 1980. A sociobiological perspective on divorce patterns of men in the United States. *Journal of Anthropological Research* 36:419.

MacLusky, N.J. and Naftolin, F. 1981. Sexual differentiation of the central nervous system. *Science* 211:1294.

MacNair, M.R., and Parker, G.A. 1978. Models of parent-offspring conflict. II. Promiscuity. *Animal Behaviour* 26:111.

Magaro, P.A. 1981. The paranoid and the schizophrenic: The case for distinct cognitive style. *Schizophrenia Bulletin* 7:632.

Mahler, M.S. 1971. A study of the separation-individuation process and its possible application to borderline phenomena in the psychoanalytic situation. *Psychoanalytic Study of the Child* 26:403.

Mahler, M.S., Pine, F., and Bergman, A. 1975. *The Psychological Birth of the Human Infant*. New York: Basic Books.

Main, M., Kaplan, N., and Cassidy, J. 1985. Security in infancy, childhood, and adulthood: A move to the level of representation. *Monographs of the Society for Research in Child Development* 50(1-2):66.

Main, M., and Weston, D.R. 1982. Avoidance of the attachment figure in infancy: Descriptions and interpretations. In *The Place of Attachment in Human Behavior*. C.M. Parkes, and J. Stevenson-Hinde, editors. New York: Basic Books.

Malinowski, B. 1927. *Sex and Repression in Savage Society*. Cleveland: Meridian.

———. 1932. *Sexual Life of Savages*, 3rd Ed. London: Routledge.

———. 1961. *Argonauts of the Western Pacific*. New York: Dutton.

Manstead, A.S.R., and Wagner, H.L. 1981. Arousal, cognition, and emotion: An appraisal of two-factor theory. *Current Psychological Reviews* 1:35.

Margolis, R., Prieto, P., Stein, L., et al. 1971. Statistical summary of 10,000 male cases using Afrodex in treatment of impotence. *Current Therapeutic Research* 13:616.

Markl, H.S., Butenandt, E., Campbell, D.T., et al. 1978. Evolution of morals? Morals of evolution?: Group report. In *Morality as a Biological Phenomenon*. G.S. Stent, editor. Berlin: Dahlem Konferenzen.

Marks, I.M. 1969. *Fears and Phobias*. New York: Academic Press.

———. 1987. *Fears, Phobias, and Rituals: Panic, Anxiety, and their Disorders*. New York: Oxford University Press.

Marler, P. 1979. Development of auditory perception in relation to vocal behavior. In *Human Ethology: Claims and Limits of a New Discipline*. M. von Cranach, K. Foppa, W. Lepenies, et al., editors. New York: Cambridge University Press.

Marmor, J. 1954. Orality in the hysterical personality. *Journal of the American Psychoanalytic Association* 1:656.

Mason, W.A. 1963. The effects of environmental restriction on the social development of rhesus monkeys. In *Primate Social Behavior*. C.H. Southwick, editor. Princeton, NJ: Van Nostrand.

———. 1979. Maternal attributes and primate cognitive development. In *Human Ethology: Claims and Limits of a New Discipline*. M. von Cranach, K. Foppa, W. Lepenies, et al., editors. New York: Cambridge University Press.

Mason, W.A., Davenport, R.K., and Menzel, E.W. 1968. Early experience and the social development of rhesus monkeys and chimpanzees. In *Early Experience and Behavior*. G. Newton, and S. Levine, editors. Springfield, MO: Charles C. Thomas.

Matas, L., Arend, R.A., and Sroufe, L.A. 1978. Continuity of adaptation in the second year: The relationship between quality of attachment and later competence. *Child Development* 49:547.

Mathews, A.M., Gelder, M.G., and Johnston, D.W. 1981. *Agoraphobia: Nature and Treatment*. New York: Guilford Press.

Mattsson, A., and Kim, S.P. 1985. Psychological factors affecting physical conditions (psychosomatic disorders). In *Comprehensive Textbook of Psychiatry*, 4th Ed. H.I. Kaplan, and B.J. Sadock, eds. Baltimore: Williams and Wilkins.

Matussek, P., and Feil, W.B. 1983. Personality attributes of depressive patients: Results of group comparisons. *Archives of General Psychiatry* 40:783.

Matussek, P., and Luks, O. 1981. Themes of endogenous and nonendogenous depressions. *Psychiatry Research* 5:235.

Mauss, M. 1954. *The Gift*. I. Cunnison, trans. London: Routledge and Kegan Paul.

Maxwell, M. 1984. *Human Evolution: A Philosophical Anthropology*. New York: Columbia University Press.

Maynard Smith, J. 1964. Group selection and kin selection. *Nature* 201:1145.

———. 1974. The theory of games and the evolution of animal conflicts. *Journal of Theoretical Biology* 47:209.

———. 1976a. Evolution and the theory of games. *American Scientist* 64:41.

———. 1976b. Group selection. *Quarterly Review of Biology* 51:277.

———. 1982a. The evolution of social behaviour—a classification of models. In *Current Problems in Sociobiology*. King's College Sociobiology Group, editors. Cambridge: Cambridge University Press.

———. 1982b. *Evolution and the Theory of Games*. Cambridge: Cambridge University Press.

———. ed. 1982c. *Evolution Now: A Century After Darwin*. San Francisco: W.H. Freeman.

Maynard Smith, J., and Parker, G.A. 1976. The logic of asymmetric contests. *Animal Behaviour* 24:159.

Maynard Smith, J., and Price, G.R. 1973. The logic of animal conflict. *Nature, London*: 246:15.

Mayr, E. 1963. *Animal Species and Evolution*. Cambridge, MA: Harvard University Press.

McCardel, J., and Murray, E.J. 1974. Non-specific factors in weekend encounter groups. *Journal of Consulting and Clinical Psychology* 42:337.

McGlashan, T. 1983a. The borderline syndrome, I: Testing three diagnostic systems for borderline. *Archives of General Psychiatry* 40:1311.

———. 1983b. The borderline syndrome, II: Is borderline a variant of schizophrenia or affective disorder? *Archives of General Psychiatry* 40:1319.

———. 1986. Schizophrenia: Psychosocial treatments and the role of psychosocial factors in its etiology and pathogenesis. In *American Psychiatric Association*

Annual Review, Vol. 5. A.J. Frances, and R.E. Hales, editors. Washington, D.C.: American Psychiatric Press.

McGuire, M.R., and Essock-Vitale, S.M. 1981. Psychiatric disorders in the context of evolutionary biology: A functional classification of behavior. *Journal of Nervous and Mental Disease* 169:672.

McGuire, M.T., Essock-Vitale, S.M., and Polsky, R.H. 1981. Psychiatric disorders in the context of evolutionary biology: An ethological model of behavioral changes associated with psychiatric disorders. *Journal of Nervous and Mental Disease* 169:687.

McGuire, M.T., and Fairbanks, L.A., eds. 1977. *Ethological Psychiatry: Psychopathology in the Context of Evolutionary Biology.* New York: Grune and Stratton.

McKinney, W.T. 1985. Separation and depression: Biological markers. In *The Psychobiology of Attachment.* M. Reite, and T. Field, editors. New York: Academic Press.

———. 1988. *Models of Mental Disorders: A New Comparative Psychiatry.* New York: Plenum.

Mead, M. 1950. *Sex and Temperament in Three Primitive Societies.* New York: Mentor Books.

———. 1967. *Male and Female: A Study of the Sexes in a Changing World.* New York: William Morrow.

Melges, F.T., and Swartz, M.S. 1989. Oscillations of attachment in borderline personality disorder. *American Journal of Psychiatry* 146:1115.

Mellen, S.L.W. 1981. *The Evolution of Love.* San Francisco: W.H. Freeman.

Metcalf, R.A., Stamps, J.A., and Krishnan, V.V. 1979. Parent-offspring conflict which is not limited by degree of kinship. *Journal of Theoretical Biology* 76:99.

Meyer-Bahlburg, H.F.L., Feldman, J.F., Cohen, P., et al. 1988. Perinatal factors in the development of gender-related play behavior: Sex hormones versus pregnancy complications. *Psychiatry* 51:260.

Michod, R.E. 1982. The theory of kin selection. *Annual Review of Ecology and Systematics* 13:23.

Milgram, S. 1961. Nationality and conformity. *Scientific American* Dec.:45.

———. 1965. Some conditions of obedience and disobedience to authority. *Human Relations* 18:57.

———. 1974. *Obedience to Authority.* New York: Harper and Row.

Miller, A. 1981. *The Drama of the Gifted Child: How Narcissistic Parents Form and Deform the Emotional Lives of Their Talented Children.* New York: Basic Books.

Mirin, S.M., Meyer, R.D., Mendelson, J.H., et al. 1980. Opiate use and sexual function. *American Journal of Psychiatry* 137:909.

Mitchell, G.D. 1968. Persistent behavior pathology in rhesus monkeys following early social isolation. *Folia Primatologica* 8:132.

———. 1970. Abnormal behavior in primates. In *Primate Behavior: Developments in Field and Laboratory Research,* Vol. 1. L.A. Rosenblum, editor. New York: Academic Press.

Mitchell, J.E., Pyle, R.L., and Eckert, E.D. 1985. Bulimia. In *American Psychiatric Association Annual Review,* Vol. 4. R.E. Hales, and A.J. Frances, editors. Washington, D.C.: American Psychiatric Press.

Mitchell, S.A. 1988. *Relational Concepts in Psychoanalysis: An Integration.* Cambridge, MA: Harvard University Press.

Miyake, K., Chen, S., and Campos, J.J. 1985. Infant temperament, mother's mode of interaction, and attachment in Japan: An interim report. *Monographs of the Society for Research in Child Development* 50(1–2):276.

Montagu, A. 1980. Introduction. In *Sociobiology Examined.* A. Montagu, editor. Oxford: Oxford University Press.

Morgan, C.L. 1890. *Animal Life and Intelligence.* Boston: Ginn.

————. 1892. The law of psychogenesis. *Mind* I:72.

Morsbach, G., and Bunting, C. 1979. Maternal recognition of their neonates' cries. *Developmental Medicine and Child Neurology* 21:178.

Morton, N.E. 1958. Empirical risks in consanguineous marriages: Birth weight, gestation time, and measurements of infants. *American Journal of Human Genetics* 10:344.

Mosher, L.R., and Gunderson, J.G. 1979. Group, family, milieu, and community support systems treatment for schizophrenia. In *Disorders of the Schizophrenic Syndrome.* L. Bellak, editor. New York: Basic Books.

Murdock, G.P. 1967. *The Ethnographic Atlas.* Pittsburgh: University of Pittsburgh Press.

Murray, R.M., and Reveley, A. 1981. The genetic contribution to the neuroses. *British Journal of Hospital Medicine* 25:185.

Mustafa, A. 1966. Female circumcision and infibulation in the Sudan. *Journal of Obstetrics and Gynaecology of the British Commonwealth* 73:302.

Myers, M.F. 1982. Homosexuality, sexual dysfunction, and incest in male identical twins. *Canadian Journal of Psychiatry* 27:144.

Neisser, U. 1982. Preface. In *Memory Observed: Remembering in Natural Contexts.* U. Neisser, ed. San Francisco: W.H. Freeman.

Nelson, M.O. 1971. The concept of God and feelings toward the parents. *Journal of Individual Psychology* 27:46.

Nelson, M.O., and Jones, E.M. 1957. An application of the Q-sort technique to the study of religious concepts. *Psychological Reports* 3:293.

Nesse, R. 1984. An evolutionary perspective on psychiatry. *Comprehensive Psychiatry* 25:575.

————. 1989. *The Evolution of Mood and Its Disorders.* Paper presented at the Human Behavior and Evolution Society First Annual Meeting. Northwestern University, Evanston, Ill. August 26.

Neumann, E. 1955. *The Great Mother: An Analysis of the Archetype.* London: Routledge and Kegan Paul.

Nicholson, N., Cole, S.G., and Rocklin, T. 1985. Conformity in the Asch situation: A comparison between contemporary British and U.S. university students. *British Journal of Social Psychology* 24:59.

Niederland, W.G. 1959a. The "miracled-up" world of Schreber's childhood. *Psychoanalytic Study of the Child* 14:383.

―――. 1959b. Schreber: Father and son. *Psycho-Analytic Quarterly* 28:151.

Noonan, K.M. 1987. Evolution: A primer for psychologists. In *Sociobiology and Psychology: Ideas, Issues and Applications*. C. Crawford, M. Smith, and D. Krebs, eds. Hillsdale, NJ: Lawrence Erlbaum.

Norton, G.R., Dorward, J., and Cox, B.J. 1986. Factors associated with panic attacks in non-clinical subjects. *Behavior Therapy* 17:239.

O'Connor, R.J. 1978. Brood reduction in birds: Selection for fratricide, infanticide and suicide? *Animal Behaviour* 26:79.

O'Connor, S.M., Vietze, P.M., Hopkins, J.B., et al. 1977. Post-partum extended maternal-infant contact: Subsequent mothering and child health. *Pediatric Research* 11:380.

Olweus, D., Mattsson, A., Schalling, D., et al. 1988. Circulating testosterone levels and aggression in adolescent males: A causal analysis. *Psychosomatic Medicine* 50:261.

Orians, G.H. 1969. On the evolution of mating systems in birds and mammals. *American Naturalist* 103:589.

Ornstein, P., ed. 1978. *The Search for the Self: Selected Writings of Heinz Kohut, 1950–1978*. New York: International Universities Press.

Overall, J.E., Hollister, L.E., and Pennington, V. 1966. Nosology of depression and differential response to drugs. *Journal of the American Medical Association* 195:946.

Owen, G. 1982. *Game Theory*, 2nd Ed. New York: Academic Press.

Panksepp, J., Herman, B., Conner, R., et al. 1978. The biology of social attachments: Opiates relieve separation distress. *Biological Psychiatry* 13:607.

Papousek, H., and Papousek, M. 1979. Early ontogeny of human social interaction: Its biological roots and social dimensions. In *Human Ethology: Claims and Limits of a New Discipline*. M. von Cranach, K. Foppa, W. Lepenies, et al., editors. New York: Cambridge University Press.

Pareto, V. 1963. *A Treatise on General Sociology*. New York: Dover Publications.

Pargament, K.I., Steele, R.E., and Tyler, F.B. 1979. Religious participation, religious motivation, and psychosocial competence. *Journal for the Scientific Study of Religion* 18:412.

Park, R.E. 1928. Human migration and the marginal man. *American Journal of Sociology* 33:881.

Parker, G. 1979a. Reported parental characteristics of agoraphobics and social phobics. *British Journal of Psychiatry* 135:555.

―――. 1979b. Parental characteristics in relation to depressive disorders. *British Journal of Psychiatry* 134:138.

―――. 1981. Parental reports of depressives: An investigation of several explanations. *Journal of Affective Disorder* 3:131.

―――. 1983. Parental "affectionless control" as an antecedent to adult depression: A risk factor delineated. *Archives of General Psychiatry* 40:956.

Parker, G.A. 1974. Assessment strategy and the evolution of fighting behaviour. *Journal of Theoretical Biology* 47:223.

———. 1982. Phenotype-limited evolutionarily stable strategies. In *Current Problems in Sociobiology*. King's College Sociobiology Group, editors. Cambridge, England: Cambridge University Press.

Parker, G.A., and MacNair, M.R. 1978. Models of parent-offspring conflict. I. Monogamy. *Animal Behaviour* 26:97.

Parkes, C.M., and Weiss, R.S. 1983. *Recovery from Bereavement*. New York: Basic Books.

Patterson, M.L. 1985. Social influence and nonverbal exchange. In *Power, Dominance, and Nonverbal Behavior*. S.L. Ellyson, and J.F. Dovidio, editors. New York: Springer-Verlag.

Peroutka, S.J., and Snyder, S.H. 1980. Relationship of neuroleptic drug effects at brain dopamine, serotonin, alpha-adrenergic, and histamine receptors to clinical potency. *American Journal of Psychiatry* 137:1518.

Perry, J., and Klerman, G. 1980. Clinical features of the borderline personality disorder. *American Journal of Psychiatry* 137:165.

Pettijohn, T.F. 1979. Attachment and separation distress in the infant guinea pig. *Developmental Psychobiology* 12:73.

Pettijohn, T.F., Wong, T.W., Ebert, P.D., et al. 1977. Alleviation of separation distress in three breeds of young dogs. *Developmental Psychobiology* 10:373.

Pfohl, B., Stangl, D.D., and Tsuang, M.T. 1983. The association between early parental loss and diagnosis in the Iowa 500. *Archives of General Psychiatry* 40:965.

Pfohl, B., Stangl, D.D., and Zimmerman, M. 1984. The implications of DSM-III personality disorders for patients with major depression. *Journal of Affective Disorders* 7:309.

Piaget, J. 1954. *The Construction of Reality in the Child*. New York: Basic Books.

———. 1978. *Behavior and Evolution*. D. Nicholson-Smith, trans. New York: Pantheon.

Pianka, E.R. 1970. On r- and K-selection. *American Naturalist* 104:592.

Pilkonis, P.A. 1988. Personality prototypes among depressives: Themes of dependency and autonomy. *Journal of Personality Disorders* 2:144.

Pilkonis, P.A., and Frank, E. 1988. Personality pathology in recurrent depression: Nature, prevalence, and relationship to treatment response. *American Journal of Psychiatry* 145:435.

Pilowsky, I., and Bassett, D. 1980. Schizophrenia and the response to facial emotions. *Comprehensive Psychiatry* 21:236.

Pilowsky, I., and Spence, N.D. 1975. Hostility and depressive illness. *Archives of General Psychiatry* 32:1154.

Pitts, F.N., and McClure, J.N. 1967. Lactate metabolism in anxiety neurosis. *New England Journal of Medicine* 227:1329.

Ploog, D. 1979. Comments on papers by Marler and Liberman. In *Human Ethology: Claims and Limits of a New Discipline*. M. von Cranach, K. Foppa, W. Lepenies, et al., editors. New York: Cambridge University Press.

Pope, H.G., Jonas, J.M., Hudson, J.I., et al. 1983. The validity of DSM-III borderline personality disorder: A phenomenologic, family history, treatment response, and long-term follow-up study. *Archives of General Psychiatry* 40:23.

Porter, R.H. 1987. Kin recognition: Functions and mediating mechanisms. In *Sociobiology and Psychology: Ideas, Issues and Applications.* C. Crawford, M. Smith, and D. Krebs, eds. Hillsdale, NJ: Lawrence Erlbaum.

Porter, R.H., Cernoch, J.M., and Balogh, R.D. 1984. Recognition of neonates by facial-visual characteristics. *Pediatrics* 74:501.

Porter, R.H., Cernoch, J.M., and McLaughlin, F.J. 1983. Maternal recognition of neonates through olfactory cues. *Physiology and Behavior* 30:151.

Potter, W.Z., Rudorfer, M.V., and Goodwin, F.K. 1987. Biological findings in bipolar disorders. In *American Psychiatric Association Annual Review,* Vol. 6. R.E. Hales, and A.J. Frances, eds. Washington, D.C.: American Psychiatric Press.

Pound, A. 1982. Attachment and maternal depression. In *The Place of Attachment in Human Behavior.* C.M. Parkes, and J. Stevenson-Hinde, editors. New York: Basic Books.

Price, J. 1967. Hypothesis: The dominance hierarchy and the evolution of mental illness. *Lancet* 2:243.

———. 1969. The ritualization of agonistic behaviour as a determinant of variation along the neuroticism/stability dimension of personality. *Proceedings of the Royal Society of Medicine* 62:1107.

———. 1972. Genetic and phylogenetic aspects of mood variation. *International Journal of Mental Health* 1:124.

Price, J., and Sloman, L. 1984. The evolutionary model of psychiatric disorder. *Archives of General Psychiatry* 41:211.

Pugh, G.E. 1977. *The Biological Origin of Human Values.* New York: Basic Books.

Rabin, A.I., Doneson, S.L., and Jentons, R.L. 1979. Studies of psychological functions in schizophrenia. In *Disorders of the Schizophrenic Syndrome.* L. Bellak, editor. New York: Basic Books.

Rachman, S. 1966. Sexual fetishism: An experimental analogue. *Psychological Record* 16:293.

Rachman, S., and Hodgson, R.J. 1968. Experimentally induced sexual fetishism: Replication and development. *Psychological Record* 18:25.

Rainey, J.M., Pohl, R.B., Williams, M., et al. 1984. A comparison of lactate and isoproterenol anxiety states. *Psychopathology* 17:74.

Raleigh, M.J., and Steklis, H.D. 1981. Effects of orbitofrontal and temporal neocortical lesions on the affiliative behavior of vervet monkeys (*Cercopithecus aethiops sabaeus*). *Experimental Neurology* 73:378.

Raleigh, M.J., Steklis, H.D., Ervin, F.R., et al. 1979. The effects of orbitofrontal lesions on the aggressive behavior of vervet monkeys (*Cercopithecus aethiops sabaeus*). *Experimental Neurology* 66:158.

Rapaport, D., Gill, M.M., and Schafer, R. 1968. *Diagnostic Psychological Testing,* Rev. Ed. New York: International Universities Press.

Raphael, B. 1983. *The Anatomy of Bereavement.* New York: Basic Books.

Rasmussen, S.A., and Tsuang, M.T. 1986. Clinical characteristics and family history in DSM-III obsessive-compulsive disorder. *American Journal of Psychiatry* 143:317.

Reich, J. 1988. DSM-III personality disorders and family history of mental illness. *Journal of Nervous and Mental Disease* 176:45.

Reich, J., and Troughton, E. 1988. Comparison of DSM-III personality disorders in recovered depressed and panic disorder patients. *Journal of Nervous and Mental Disease* 176:300.

Reite, M., Short, R., Seiler, C., et al. 1981. Attachment, loss and depression. *Journal of Child Psychology and Psychiatry* 22:141.

Resko, J.A. 1975. Fetal hormones and their effect on the differentiation of the CNS in primates. *Federation Proceedings* 34:1650.

Reynolds, V., and Tanner, R.E.S. 1983. *The Biology of Religion.* London: Longman.

Richards, R.J. 1987. *Darwin and the Emergence of Evolutionary Theories of Mind and Behavior.* Chicago: University of Chicago Press.

Richerson, P.J., and Boyd, R. 1989. The role of evolved predispositions in cultural evolution: Or, human sociobiology meets Pascal's wager. *Ethology and Sociobiology* 10:195.

Ricks, D.M., and Wing, L. 1975. Language, communication, and the use of symbols in normal and autistic children. *Journal of Autism and Childhood Schizophrenia* 5:191.

Rieff, P. 1966. *The Triumph of the Therapeutic: Uses of Faith after Freud.* New York: Harper and Row.

Rifkin, A., Klein, D.F., Dillon, D., et al. 1981. Blockade by imipramine or desimipramine of panic induced by sodium lactate. *American Journal of Psychiatry* 138:676.

Rizley, R. 1978. Depression and distortion in the attribution of causality. *Journal of Abnormal Psychology* 87:32.

Rizzuto, A. 1976. Freud, God, and the Devil and the theory of object representations. *International Review of Psycho-Analysis* 31:165.

———. 1979. *The Birth of the Living God: A Psychoanalytic Study.* Chicago: University of Chicago Press.

Roberts, A.H. 1964. Housebound housewives: A follow-up study of a phobic anxiety state. *British Journal of Psychiatry* 110:191.

Robin, A.A., Copas, J.B., Jack, A.B., et al. 1988. Reshaping the psyche: The concurrent improvement in appearance and mental state after rhinoplasty. *British Journal of Psychiatry* 152:539.

Robinson, D.N. 1979. *Systems of Modern Psychology: A Critical Sketch.* New York: Columbia University Press.

Rohrbaugh, J.B. 1979. *Women: Psychology's Puzzle.* New York: Basic Books.

Rose, R.M., Gordon, T.P., and Bernstein, I.S. 1971. Plasma testosterone levels in the male rhesus: Influences of sexual and social stimuli. *Science* 178:643.

———. 1972. Sexual and social influence on testosterone secretion in the rhesus. *Psychosomatic Medicine* 34:473.

Rose, R.M., Holaday, J.W., and Bernstein, I.S. 1971. Plasma testosterone, dominance rank, and aggressive behavior in rhesus monkeys. *Nature* 231:366.

Rosenbaum, J.F., Biederman, J., Gersten, M., et al. 1988. Behavioral inhibition in children of parents with panic disorder and agoraphobia: A controlled study. *Archives of General Psychiatry* 45:463.

Rosenblatt, J.S. 1976. Stages in the early behavioural development of altricial young of selected species of non-primate mammals. In *Growing Points in Ethology*. P.P.G. Bateson, and R.A. Hinde, editors. New York: Cambridge University Press.

Rosenblum, L.A. 1971. The ontogeny of mother-infant relations in macaques. In *The Ontogeny of Vertebrate Behavior*. H. Moltz, editor. New York: Academic Press.

Rosenthal, T.L., Akiskal, H.S., Scott-Strauss, A., et al. 1981. Familial and developmental factors in characterological depressions. *Journal of Affective Disorders* 3:183.

Ross, E.D., and Rush, A.J. 1981. Diagnosis and neuroanatomical correlates of depression in brain-damaged patients. *Archives of General Psychiatry* 38:1344.

Roth, L.H. 1971. Territoriality and homosexuality in a male prison population. *American Journal of Orthopsychiatry* 41:510.

Roth, M. 1959. The phobic anxiety-depersonalization syndrome. *Proceedings of the Royal Society of Medicine* 52:587.

———. 1960. The phobic anxiety-depersonalization syndrome and some general aetiological problems in psychiatry. *Journal of Neuropsychiatry* 1:293.

Rounsaville, B.J., Weissman, M.M., Kleber, H., et al. 1982. Heterogeneity of psychiatric diagnosis in treated opiate addicts. *Archives of General Psychiatry* 32:162.

Roy-Byrne, P.P., Geraci, M., and Uhde, T.W. 1986. Life events and the onset of panic disorder. *American Journal of Psychiatry* 143:1424.

Rozin, P., and Kalat, J.W. 1971. Specific hungers and poison avoidance as adaptive specialization of learning. *Psychological Review* 78:459.

Rubin, R.T., Reinisch, J.M., and Haskett, R.F. 1981. Postnatal gonadal steroid effects on human behavior. *Science* 211:1318.

Rubenstein, C.M., and Shaver, P. 1980. Loneliness in two northeastern cities. In *The Anatomy of Loneliness*. J. Hartog, J.R. Audy, and Y.A. Cohen, editors. New York: International Universities Press.

Rudden, M., Sweeney, J., Frances, A., et al. 1983. A comparison of delusional disorders in women and men. *American Journal of Psychiatry* 140:1575.

Ruse, M. 1980. Charles Darwin and group selection. *Annals of Science* 37:615.

———. 1987. Sociobiology and knowledge: Is evolutionary epistemology a viable option? In *Sociobiology and Psychology: Ideas, Issues and Applications*. C. Crawford, M. Smith, and D. Krebs, eds. Hillsdale, N.J. Lawrence Erlbaum.

Rushton, J.P., Russell, R.J.H., and Wells, P.A. 1984. Genetic similarity theory: Beyond kin recognition. *Behavior Genetics* 14:179.

Russell, M.J. 1976. Human olfactory communication. *Nature* 260:520.

Russell, M.J., Mendelsohn, T., and Peeke, H.V.S. 1983. Mother's identification of their infant's odors. *Ethology and Sociobiology* 4:29.

Rutter, M. 1972. *Maternal Deprivation Reassessed.* New York: Penguin.

Sade, D.S. 1968. Inhibition of son-mother mating among free-ranging Rhesus monkeys. *Science and Psychoanalysis* 12:18.

Sadock, V.A. 1985. Special areas of interest. In *Comprehensive Textbook of Psychiatry,* 4th Ed. H.I. Kaplan, and B.J. Sadock, editors. Baltimore: Williams and Wilkins.

Saghir, M.T., and Robins, E. 1973. *Male and Female Homosexuality: A Comprehensive Investigation.* Baltimore: Williams and Wilkins.

Sagi, A., Lamb, M.E., Lewkowicz, K.S. et al. 1985. Security of infant-mother, -father, and -metapelet attachments among kibbutz-reared Israeli children. *Monographs of the Society for Research in Child Development* 50(1–2):257.

Sahlins, M.D. 1976. *The Use and Abuse of Biology: An Anthropological Critique of Sociobiology.* Ann Arbor: University of Michigan Press.

Sakurai, M.M. 1975. Small group cohesiveness and detrimental conformity. *Sociometry* 38:340.

Salk, L. 1973. The role of the heartbeat in the relations between mother and infant. *Scientific American* 228:24.

Salzen, E.A. 1979. Social attachment and a sense of security. In *Human Ethology: Claims and Limits of a New Discipline.* M. von Cranach, K. Foppa, W. Lepenies, et al., editors. New York: Cambridge University Press.

Sameroff, A.J., Seifer, R., and Zax, M. 1982. Early development of children at risk of emotional disorder. *Monographs of the Society for Research in Child Development* 47(7):1.

Sartorius, N., Jablensky, A., and Shapiro, R. 1978. Cross-cultural differences in the short-term prognosis of schizophrenic psychoses. *Schizophrenia Bulletin* 4:102.

Schachter, S. 1964. The interaction of cognitive and physiological determinants of emotion state. In *Advances in Experimental Social Psychology,* Vol. 1. L. Berkowitz, editor. New York: Academic Press.

Schachter, S., and Singer, J.E. 1962. Cognitive, social, and physiological determinants of emotional state. *Psychological Review* 69:379.

Schachter, S., and Wheeler, L. 1962. Epinephrine, chlorpromazine, and amusement. *Journal of Abnormal and Social Psychology* 65:121.

Schaffer, H.R., and Emerson, P.E. 1964. The development of social attachments in infancy. *Monographs of the Society for Research in Child Development* 29(3):1.

Schaller, G.B. 1963. *The Mountain Gorilla: Ecology and Behavior.* Chicago: University of Chicago Press.

Schapira, K., Kerr, T.A., and Roth, M. 1970. Phobias and affective illness. *British Journal of Psychiatry* 117:25.

Schiavi, R.C. 1981. Male erectile disorders. *Annual Review of Medicine* 32:509.

Schmookler, A.B. 1984. *The Parable of the Tribes: The Problem of Power in Social Evolution*. Boston: Houghton Mifflin.

Schuldberg, D., French, C., Stone, B.L., et al. 1988. Creativity and schizotypal traits: Creativity test scores and perceptual aberration, magical ideation, and impulsive nonconformity. *Journal of Nervous and Mental Disease* 176:648.

Schull, W.J. 1958. Empirical risks in consanguineous marriages: Sex ratio, malformation, and viability. *American Journal of Human Genetics* 10:294.

Schulz, S.C., Schulz, P.M., and Wilson, W.H. 1988. Medication treatment of schizotypal personality disorder. *Journal of Personality Disorders* 2:1.

Schumacher, M., and Balthazart, J. 1985. Sexual differentiation is a biphasic process in mammals and birds. In *Neurobiology*. R. Gilles, and J. Balthazart, editors. New York: Springer-Verlag.

Schumacher, M., Legros, J.J., and Balthazart, J. 1987. Steroid hormones, behavior and sexual dimorphism in animals and men: The nature-nurture controversy. *Experimental and Clinical Endocrinology* 90:129.

Seemanova, E. 1971. A study of children of incestuous matings. *Human Heredity* 21:108.

Segal, N.L. 1988. Cooperation, competition, and altruism in human twinships: A sociobiological approach. In *Sociobiological Perspectives on Human Development*. K.B. MacDonald, ed. New York: Springer-Verlag.

Seligman, M.E. 1975. *Helplessness: On Depression, Development, and Death*. San Francisco: W.H. Freeman.

Sermat, V. 1980. Some situational and personality correlates of loneliness. In *The Anatomy of Loneliness*. J. Hartog, J.R. Audy, and Y.A. Cohen, editors. New York: International Universities Press.

Shea, M.T., Glass, D.R., Pilkonis, P.A., et al. 1987. Frequency and implications of personality disorders in a sample of depressed outpatients. *Journal of Personality Disorders* 1:27.

Shear, M.K., and Fyer, M.R. 1988. Biological and psychopathologic findings in panic disorder. In *American Psychiatric Press Review of Psychiatry*, Vol. 7. A.J. Frances, and R.E. Hales, eds. Washington, D.C.: American Psychiatric Press.

Sheehan, D.V., Ballenger, J., and Jacobsen, G. 1980. Treatment of endogenous anxiety. *Archives of General Psychiatry* 37:51.

Sheehy, M., Goldsmith, I., and Charles, E. 1980. A comparative study of borderline patients in a psychiatric outpatient clinic. *American Journal of Psychiatry* 137:1374.

Sheldon, H. 1988. Childhood sexual abuse in adult female psychotherapy referrals: Incidence and implications for treatment. *British Journal of Psychiatry* 152:107.

Shepher, J. 1983. *Incest: A Biosocial View*. New York: Academic Press.

Shepherd, G. 1978. The Omani Xanith. *Man* 13:663.

Sherif, M. 1937. An experimental approach to the study of attitudes. *Sociometry* 1:90.

———. 1966. *Group Conflict and Cooperation: Their Social Psychology*. London: Routledge and Kegan Paul.

Sherrod, L.R. 1981. Issues in cognitive-perceptual development: The special case of social stimuli. In *Infant Social Cognition*. M.E. Lamb, and L.R. Sherrod, editors. Hillsdale, NJ: Erlbaum.

Short, R.V. 1976. The evolution of human reproduction. *Proceedings of the Royal Society* (ser. B) 195:3.

Shubik, M. 1982. *Game Theory in the Social Sciences: Concepts and Solutions*. Cambridge, MA: MIT Press.

Siegman, A.W. 1961. An empirical investigation of the psychoanalytic theory of religious behavior. *Journal for the Scientific Study of Religion* 1:74.

Siever, L.J., and Gunderson, J.G. 1983. The search for schizotypal personality: Historical origins and current status. *Comprehensive Psychiatry* 24:199.

Siever, L.J., and Klar, H. 1986. A review of DSM-III criteria for the personality disorders. In *American Psychiatric Association Annual Review*, Vol. 5. A.J. Frances, and R.E. Hales, editors. Washington, D.C.: American Psychiatric Press.

Silk, J.B., and Boyd, R. 1983. Cooperation, competition, and mate choice in matrilineal macaque groups. In *Social Behavior of Female Vertebrates*. S.K. Wasser, editor. New York: Academic Press.

Silverman, I. 1987. Race, race differences, and race relations: Perspectives from psychology and sociobiology. In *Sociobiology and Psychology: Ideas, Issues and Applications*. C. Crawford, M. Smith, and D. Krebs, eds. Hillsdale, NJ: Lawrence Erlbaum.

Simpson, G.G. 1953a. *The Major Features of Evolution*. New York: Columbia University Press.

———. 1953b. The Baldwin effect. *Evolution* 7:110.

Slap, G.W., and Levine, F.J. 1978. On hybrid concepts in psychoanalysis. *Psychoanalytic Quarterly* 67:499.

Slater, E., and Roth, M. 1969. *Clinical Psychiatry*, 3rd Ed. London: Bailliere, Tindall and Cassell.

Slavin, M.O. 1985. The origins of psychic conflict and the adaptive function of repression: An evolutionary biological view. *Psychoanalysis and Contemporary Thought* 8:407.

Slavin, M.O., and Kriegman, D. 1988. Freud, biology, and sociobiology. *American Psychologist* 43:658.

Sloman, L. 1981. Intrafamilial struggles for power: An ethological perspective. *International Journal of Family Psychiatry* 2:13.

———. 1983. Inclusive fitness, altruism and family adaptation. *Canadian Journal of Psychiatry* 28:18.

Sloman, L., Konstantareas, M., and Dunham, D.W. 1979. The adaptive role of maladaptive neurosis. *Biological Psychiatry* 14:961.

Smith, M.S. 1988. Research in developmental sociobiology: Parenting and family behavior. In *Sociobiological Perspectives on Human Development*. K.B. MacDonald, ed. New York: Springer-Verlag.

Smith, P.K. 1979. The ontogeny of fear in children. In *Fear in Animals and Man*. W. Sluckin, editor. London: Van Nostrand.

Smith, T.W., O'Keefe, J.L., and Jenkins, M. 1988. Dependency and self-criticism:

Correlates of depression or moderators of the effects of stressful events? *Journal of Personality Disorders* 2:160.

Snaith, R.P. 1968. A clinical investigation of phobias. *British Journal of Psychiatry* 114:673.

Snow, C. 1972. Mother's speech to children learning language. *Child Development* 43:549.

Snyder, S.H., and Largent, B.L. 1989. Receptor mechanisms in antipsychotic drug action: Focus on sigma receptors. *Journal of Neuropsychiatry* 1:7.

Soloff, P.H., George, A., and Nathan, R.S. 1982. The dexamethasone suppression test in patients with borderline personality. *American Journal of Psychiatry* 139:1621.

Soloff, P.H., and Millward, J.W. 1983. Psychiatric disorders in the families of borderline patients. *Archives of General Psychiatry* 40:37.

Soloff, P.H. and Ulrich, R. 1981. The diagnostic interview for borderlines: A replication study. *Archives of General Psychiatry* 38:686.

Sowell, T. 1985. *Marxism.* New York: Morrow.

Spencer, H. 1851. *Social Statics: Or, the Conditions Essential to Human Happiness Specified, and the First of Them Developed.* London: Chapman.

Spencer-Booth, Y., and Hinde, R.A. 1967. The effects of separating rhesus monkeys from their mothers for six days. *Journal of Child Psychology and Psychiatry* 7:179.

———. 1971a. Effects of brief separations from mothers during infancy on behaviour of rhesus monkeys 6–24 months later. *Journal of Child Psychology and Psychiatry* 12:157.

———. 1971b. Effects of six days' separation from mother on 18- to 32-week-old rhesus monkeys. *Animal Behavior* 19:174.

Sperber, M.A., and Jarvik, L.F. 1976. *Psychiatry and Genetics.* New York: Basic Books.

Spilka, B. 1977. Utilitarianism and personal faith. *Journal of Psychology and Theology* 5:226.

Spiro, M.E. 1958. *Children of the Kibbutz.* Cambridge: MA: Harvard University Press.

Spiro, M.E., and D'Andrade, R.G. 1958. A cross-cultural study of some religious beliefs. *American Anthropologist* 60:456.

Spitz, R.A. 1965. *The First Year of Life.* New York: International Universities Press.

Spitzer, R.L., Endicott, J., and Gibbon, A.M. 1979. Crossing the border into borderline personality and borderline schizophrenia: The development of criteria. *Archives of General Psychiatry* 36:17.

Sroufe, L.A. 1983. Infant-caregiver attachment and patterns of adaptation in preschool: The roots of maladaptation and competence. *Minnesota Symposium in Child Psychology* 16:41.

Sroufe, L.A., Schork, E., Motti, E., et al. 1984. The role of affect in emerging social competence. In *Emotion, Cognition and Behavior.* C. Izard, J. Kagan, and R. Zajonc, editors. New York: Cambridge University Press.

Stamps, J.A., Metcalf, R.A., and Krishnan, V.V. 1978. A genetic analysis of parent-offspring conflict. *Journal of Behavioral Ecology and Sociobiology* 3:369.

Stearns, S.C. 1977. The evolution of life history traits: A critique of the theory and a review of the data. *Annual Review of Ecological Systems* 8:145.

———. 1982. The role of development in the evolution of life histories. In *Evolution and Development.* J.T. Bonner, ed. New York: Springer-Verlag.

Steinman, D.L., Wincze, J.P., Sakheim, K., et al. 1981. A comparison of male and female patterns of sexual arousal. *Archives of Sexual Behavior* 10:529.

Stent, G.S., ed. 1978a. *Morality as a Biological Phenomenon.* Berlin: Dahlem Konferenzen.

———. 1978b. Introduction: The limits of the naturalistic approach to morality. In *Morality as a Biological Phenomenon.* G.S. Stent, editor. Berlin: Dahlem Konferenzen.

Stern, C. 1960. *Principles of Human Genetics,* 2nd Ed. San Francisco: W.H. Freeman.

Stern, D.N. 1977. *The First Relationship: Infant and Mother.* Cambridge, MA: Harvard University Press.

———. 1985. *The Interpersonal World of the Infant: A View from Psychoanalysis and Developmental Psychology.* New York: Basic Books.

Stern, D.N., MacKain, K., and Spieker, S. 1982. Intonation contours as signals in maternal speech to prelinguistic infants. *Developmental Psychology* 18:727.

Stevens, A. 1982. *Archetypes: A Natural History of the Self.* New York: Quill.

Stolorow, R. 1976. Psychoanalytic reflections on client-centered therapy in the light of modern conceptions of narcissism. *Psychotherapy: Theory, Research and Practice* 13:26.

Stone, M.H. 1980. *The Borderline Syndromes: Constitution, Personality, and Adaptation.* New York: McGraw-Hill.

———. 1981. Borderline syndromes: A consideration of subtypes and an overview, directions for research. *Psychiatric Clinics of North America* 4:3.

Strauss, J.S., and Carpenter, W.T. 1981. *Schizophrenia.* New York: Plenum.

Struhsaker, T.T. 1971. Social behaviour of mother and infant vervet monkeys (*Cercopithecus aethiops*). *Animal Behavior* 19:233.

Strunk, O. 1959. Perceived relationships between parental and deity concepts. *Psychological Newsletter* 10:222.

Sugiyama, Y. 1967. Social organization of Hanuman langurs. In *Social Communication among Primates.* S. Altman, editor. Chicago: University of Chicago Press.

———. 1969. Social behavior of chimpanzees in the Budongo Forest, Uganda. *Primates* 10:197.

Sulloway, F.J. 1979. *Freud, Biologist of the Mind: Beyond the Psychoanalytic Legend.* New York: Basic Books.

Suomi, S.J., Collins, M.L., and Harlow, H.F. 1973. Effects of permanent separation from mother on infant monkeys. *Developmental Psychology* 9:376.

Suomi, S.J., Kramer, G.W., Baysinger, C.M., et al. 1981. Inherited and experimental factors associated with individual differences in anxious behavior displayed by rhesus monkeys. In *Anxiety: New Research and Changing Concepts*. D.F. Klein, and J. Rabkin, eds. New York: Raven Press.

Surtees, P.G., Miller, P.M., Ingham, J.G., et al. 1986. Life events and the onset of affective disorder: A longitudinal general population study. *Journal of Affective Disorders* 10:37.

Suzuki, A. 1971. Carnivory and cannibalism observed among forest-living chimpanzees. *Journal of the Anthropological Society of Nippon* 79:30.

Swenson, C. 1989. Kernberg and Linehan: Two approaches to the borderline patient. *Journal of Personality Disorders* 3:26.

Swift, W.J., Andrews, D., and Barklage, N.E. 1986. The relationship between affective disorder and eating disorders: A review of the literature. *American Journal of Psychiatry* 143:290.

Symons, D. 1979. *The Evolution of Human Sexuality*. New York: Oxford University Press.

———. 1987. If we're all Darwinians, what's all the fuss about? In *Sociobiology and Psychology: Ideas, Issues and Applications*. C. Crawford, M. Smith, and D. Krebs, eds. Hillsdale, NJ: Lawrence Erlbaum.

Tajfel, H. 1970. Experiments in intergroup discrimination. *Scientific American* Nov.:96.

———. 1974. Social identity and intergroup behaviour. *Social Science Information* 13:65.

———., ed. 1978. *Differentiation Between Social Groups: Studies in the Social Psychology of Intergroup Relations*. London: Academic Press.

———. 1979. Human intergroup conflict: Useful and less useful forms of analysis. In *Human Ethology: Claims and Limits of a New Discipline*. M. von Cranach, K. Foppa, W. Lepenies, et al., editors. New York: Cambridge University Press.

———. 1981. *Human Groups and Social Categories: Studies in Social Psychology*. London: Cambridge University Press.

———. 1982. Social psychology of intergroup relations. *Annual Review of Psychology* 33:1.

Tajfel, H., and Billig, M. 1974. Familiarity and categorization in intergroup behavior. *Journal of Experimental Social Psychology* 10:159.

Talmon, G.Y. 1964. Mate selection in collective settlements. *American Sociological Review* 29:408.

Tantam, D. 1988a. Lifelong eccentricity and social isolation: I. Psychiatric, social, and forensic aspects. *British Journal of Psychiatry* 153:777.

———. 1988b. Lifelong eccentricity and social isolation: II. Asperger's syndrome or schizoid personality disorder? *British Journal of Psychiatry* 153:783.

Tavris, C., and Sadd, S. 1975. *The Redbook Report on Female Sexuality*. New York: Dell.

Teleki, G. 1973. *The Predatory Behavior of Wild Chimpanzees*. Lewishburg, PA: Bucknell University Press.

Tennant, C., Bebbington, P., and Hurry, J. 1980. Parental death in childhood and risk of adult depressive disorders: A review. *Psychological Medicine* 10:289.

Tennant, C., Smith, A., Bebbington, P., et al. 1981. Parental loss in childhood. *Archives of General Psychiatry* 38:309.

Thomas, J.M. 1932. Fragments of a schizophrenic's "Virgin Mary" delusions. *American Journal of Psychiatry* 12:285.

Thompson, E.A. 1982. Gene competition without selection. In *Current Problems in Sociobiology*. King's College Sociobiology Group, editors. Cambridge: Cambridge University Press.

Thornhill, N.W., and Thornhill, R. 1987. Evolutionary theory and rules of mating and marriage pertaining to relatives. In *Sociobiology and Psychology: Ideas, Issues and Applications*. C. Crawford, M. Smith, and D. Krebs, eds. Hillsdale, NJ: Lawrence Erlbaum.

Thornhill, R., and Thornhill, N.W. 1983. Human rape: An evolutionary analysis. *Ethology and Sociobiology* 4:137.

———. 1987. Human rape: The strengths of the evolutionary perspective. In *Sociobiology and Psychology: Ideas, Issues and Applications*. C. Crawford, M. Smith, and D. Krebs, eds. Hillsdale, NJ: Lawrence Erlbaum.

Thyer, B.A., Nesse, R.M., Cameron, O.G., et al. 1985. Agoraphobia: A test of the separation anxiety hypothesis. *Behavior Research and Therapy* 23:75.

Tiger, L. 1979. *Optimism: The Biology of Hope*. New York: Simon and Schuster.

———. 1984. *Men in Groups*, 2nd Ed. New York: Marion Boyars.

Tiger, L., and Fox, R. 1971. *The Imperial Animal*. Toronto: McClelland and Stewart.

Tinbergen, W.A., and Tinbergen, N. 1972. Early childhood autism: An ethological approach. *Zeitschrift fur Tierpsychologie* (suppl.) 10:1.

Tollison, C.D., and Adams, H.E. 1979. *Sexual Disorders: Treatment, Theory, and Research*. New York: Gardner Press.

Tolpin, P.H. 1983. A change in the self: The development and transformation of an idealizing transference. *International Journal of Psychoanalysis* 64:461.

Tooby, J., and Cosmides, L. 1989. Evolutionary psychology and the generation of culture, Part I. Theoretical considerations. *Ethology and Sociobiology* 10:29.

Torrey, E.F. 1979. Epidemiology. In *Disorders of the Schizophrenic Syndrome*. L. Bellack, editor. New York: Basic Books.

Townsend, J.M. 1989. Mate selection criteria: A pilot study. *Ethology and Sociobiology* 10:241.

Trevarthen, C. 1979. Instincts for human understanding and cultural cooperation: Their development in infancy. In *Human Ethology: Claims and Limits of a New Discipline*. M. von Cranach, K. Foppa, W. Lepenies, et al., editors. New York: Cambridge University Press.

Trimingham, J.S. 1949. *Islam in the Sudan*. London: Oxford University Press.

Trivers, R.L. 1971. The evolution of reciprocal altruism. *Quarterly Review of Biology* 46:35.

———. 1972. Parental investment and sexual selection. In *Sexual Selection and the Descent of Man*. B. Campbell, editor. Chicago: Aldine.

———. 1974. Parent-offspring conflict. *American Zoologist* 14:249.

———. 1981. Sociobiology and politics. In *Sociobiology and Human Politics*. E. White, editor. Lexington, MA: Lexington Books.

———. 1985. *Social Evolution*. Menlo Park, CA.: Benjamin Cummings.

Trowell, J. 1982. Effects of obstetric management on the mother-child relationship. In *The Place of Attachment in Human Behavior.* C.M. Parkes, and J. Stevenson-Hinde, editors. New York: Basic Books.

Tsuang, M.T., Faraone, S.V., and Fleming, J.A. 1985. Familial transmission of major affective disorders: Is there evidence supporting the distinction between unipolar and bipolar disorders? *British Journal of Psychiatry* 146:268.

Tsumori, A. 1967. Newly acquired behavior and social interactions of Japanese monkeys. In *Social Communication among Primates.* S.A. Altmann, editor. Chicago: University of Chicago Press.

Turiel, E. 1978. The development of moral concepts. In *Morality as a Biological Phenomenon.* G.S. Stent, editor. Berlin: Dahlem Konferenzen.

Tyrer, P., Candy, J., and Kelly, D. 1973. Phenelzine in phobic anxiety: A controlled trial. *Psychopharmacologia* 32:237.

Tyrer, P., and Steinberg, D. 1975. Symptomatic treatment of agoraphobia and social phobias: A followup. *British Journal of Psychiatry* 127:163.

Vadher, A., and Ndetei, D.M. 1981. Life events and depression in a Kenyan setting. *British Journal of Psychiatry* 139:134.

Vaillant, G.E. 1975. Socipathy as a human process: A viewpoint. *Archives of General Psychiatry* 32:178.

Valins, S. 1966. Cognitive effects of false heart-rate feedback. *Journal of Personality and Social Psychology* 4:400.

van den Berghe, P.L. 1980. Incest and exogamy, a sociobiological reconsideration. *Ethology and Sociobiology* 1:151.

———. 1983. Human incest avoidance: Culture in nature. *Behavioral and Brain Sciences* 6:91.

———. 1987. Incest taboos and avoidance: Some African applications. In *Sociobiology and Psychology: Ideas, Issues and Applications.* C. Crawford, M. Smith, and D. Krebs, eds. Hillsdale, NJ: Lawrence Erlbaum.

Verghese, A., John, J.K., Rajkumar, S., et al. 1989. Factors associated with the course and outcome of schizophrenia in India: Results of a two-year multi-centre follow-up study. *British Journal of Psychiatry* 154:499.

Vergote, A. 1988. *Guilt and Desire: Religious Attitudes and their Pathological Derivatives.* M.H. Wood, trans. New Haven: Yale University Press.

Vergote, A., Tamayo, A., Pasquali, L., et al. 1969. Concept of God and parental images. *Journal for the Scientific Study of Religion* 8:79.

Vernon, G.M. 1968. The religious nones: A neglected category. *Journal for the Scientific Study of Religion* 7:219.

Vitz, P.C. 1988. *Sigmund Freud's Christian Unconscious.* New York: Guilford Press.

Voland, E. 1984. Human sex-ratio manipulation: Historical data from a German parish. *Journal of Human Evolution* 13:99.

Volkan, V. 1970. Typical findings in pathological grief. *Psychiatric Quarterly* 44:231.

———. 1976. *Primitive Internalized Object Relations.* New York: International Universities Press.

Waddington, C.H. 1953a. Genetic assimilation of an acquired character. *Evolution* 7:118.

————. 1953b. The Baldwin effect, genetic assimilation, and homeostasis. *Evolution* 7:386.

Wade, M.J. 1978. A critical review of the models of group selection. *Quarterly Review of Biology* 53:101.

Wallach, M.A., and Wallach, L. 1983. *Psychology's Sanction for Selfishness: The Error of Egotism in Theory and Therapy.* San Francisco: W.H. Freeman.

Wallerstein, J., and Kelly, J.B. 1980. *Surviving the Breakup.* New York: Basic Books.

Wallerstein, R.S. 1981. The bipolar self: Discussion of alternative perspectives. *Journal of the American Psychoanalytic Association* 29:377.

————. 1983. Self psychology and "classical" psychoanalytic psychology: The nature of their relationship. *Psychoanalysis and Contemporary Thought* 6:553.

————. 1985. How does self psychology differ in practice? *International Journal of Psychoanalysis* 66:391.

Warner, R. 1978. The diagnosis of antisocial and hysterical personality disorders: An example of sex bias. *Journal of Nervous and Mental Disease* 166:839.

————. 1983. Recovery from schizophrenia in the third world. *Psychiatry* 46:197.

Washburn, S.L., and DeVore, I. 1961. The social life of baboons. *Scientific American* 204(6):62.

Waters, E., Matas, L., and Sroufe, L.A. 1975. Infants' wariness to an approaching stranger. *Child Development* 46:348.

Waters, E., Wippman, J., and Sroufe, L.A. 1979. Attachment, positive affect, and competence in the peer group: Two studies in construct validation. *Child Development* 50:821.

Watson, J.S. 1971. Cognitive-perceptual development in infancy: Setting for the seventies. *Merrill-Palmer Quarterly* 17:139.

Watson, S.J., Khachaturian, H., Lewis, M.E., et al. 1986. Chemical neuroanatomy as a basis for biological psychiatry. In *American Handbook of Psychiatry,* 2nd Ed., Vol. 8. *Biological Psychiatry.* P.A. Berger, and H.K.H. Brodie, editors. New York: Basic Books.

Watt, J.A.G. 1985a. Hearing and premorbid personality in paranoid states. *American Journal of Psychiatry* 142:1453.

————. 1985b. The relationship of paranoid states to schizophrenia. *American Journal of Psychiatry* 142:1456.

Waxler, N.E. 1979. Is outcome for schizophrenia better in nonindustrialized societies?: The case of Sri Lanka. *Journal of Nervous and Mental Disease* 167:144.

Wehr, T.A., Sack, D.A., Rosenthal, N.E., et al. 1987. Sleep and biological rhythms in bipolar illness. In *American Psychiatric Association Annual Review,* Vol. 6. R.E. Hales, and A.J. Frances, editors. Washington, D.C.: American Psychiatric Press.

Weinberg, K.S. 1955. *Incest Behavior.* New York: Citadel Press.

Weinberger, D.R., Berman, K.F., and Illowsky, B.P. 1988. Physiological dysfunction of dorsolateral prefrontal cortex in schizophrenia: III. A new cohort and evidence for a monoaminergic mechanism. *Archives of General Psychiatry* 45:609.

Weinberger, D.R., and Kleinman, J.E. 1986. Observations on the brain in schizophrenia. In *American Psychiatric Association Annual Review,* Vol. 6. A.J. Frances, and R.E. Hales, editors. Washington, D.C.: American Psychiatric Press.

Weinrich, J.D. 1980. Toward a sociobiological theory of the emotions. In *Emotion: Theory, Research, and Experience,* Vol. I: *Theories of Emotion.* R. Plutchik, and H. Kellerman, eds. New York: Academic Press.

Weintraub, M., Segal, R.M., and Beck, A.T. 1974. An investigation of cognition and affect in the depressive experiences of normal men. *Journal of Consulting and Clinical Psychology* 42:911.

Weisfeld, G.E., and Billings, R.L. 1988. Observations on adolesence. In *Sociobiological Perspectives on Human Development.* K.B. MacDonald, ed. New York: Springer-Verlag.

Weiss, R.S. 1982. Attachment in adult life. In *The Place of Attachment in Human Behavior.* C.M. Parkes, and J. Stevenson-Hinde, editors, New York: Basic Books.

Weissman, M.M., Gershon, E.S., Kidd, K.K., et al. 1984. Psychiatric disorders in the relatives of probands with affective disorders. *Archives of General Psychiatry* 41:13.

Weissman, M.M., Klerman, G.L., and Paykel, E.S. 1971. Clinical evaluation of hostility in depression. *American Journal of Psychiatry* 128:261.

Weissman, M.M., Leckman, J.F., Merikangas, K.R., et al. 1984. Depression and anxiety disorders in parents and children: Results from the Yale family study. *Archives of General Psychiatry* 41:845.

Weller, M.P.I. 1988. Hysterical behaviour in patriarchal communities: Four cases, one with Ganser-like symptoms. *British Journal of Psychiatry* 152:687.

Wender, P.H., Rosenthal, D., Kety, S.S., et al. 1974. Cross-fostering: A research strategy for clarifying the role of genetic and experiental factors in the etiology of schizophrenia. *Archives of General Psychiatry* 30:121.

Wenegrat, B. 1984. *Sociobiology and Mental Disorder: A New View.* Menlo Park, CA: Addison-Wesley.

———. 1989. Religious cult membership: A sociobiologic model. In *Cults and New Religious Movements. A Report of the American Psychiatric Association.* M. Galanter, editor. Washington, D.C.: American Psychiatric Press.

———. 1990. *The Divine Archetype: The Sociobiology and Psychology of Religion.* Lexington, MA: Lexington Books.

West-Eberhard, M.J. 1978. Temporary queens in *Metapolybia* wasps: Nonreproductive helpers without altruism? *Science* 200:441.

Westermarck, E.A. 1921. *The History of Human Marriage,* 5th Ed. London: Macmillan.

———. 1926. *A Short History of Marriage.* New York: Macmillan.

————. 1934a. Recent theories of exogamy. *Sociological Review* 26:22.

————. 1934b. *Three Essays on Sex and Marriage.* London: Macmillan.

Whittaker, J.O., and Meade, R.D. 1967. Social pressure in the modification and distortion of judgment: A cross-cultural study. *International Journal of Psychology* 2:109.

Whyte, M.K. 1978. Cross-cultural codes dealing with the relative status of women. *Ethnology* 17:211.

Wikan, U. 1977. Man becomes woman: Transsexualism in Oman as a key to gender roles. *Man* 12:304.

————. 1978. The Omani Xanith. *Man* 13:667.

Wiley, R.H. 1973. Territoriality and non-random mating in sage grouse. *Animal Behaviour Monographs* 6:85.

Williams, G.C. 1966. *Adaptation and Selection.* Princeton, NJ: Princeton University Press.

————. 1975. *Sex and Evolution.* Princeton, NJ: Princeton University Press.

Williams, S.L. 1987. On anxiety and phobia. *Journal of Anxiety Disorders* 1:161.

————. 1988. Addressing misconceptions about phobia, anxiety, and self-efficacy: A reply to Marks. *Journal of Anxiety Disorders* 2:277.

Wilson, D.S. 1979. Structured demes and trait-group variation. *American Naturalist* 113:606.

————. 1980. *The Natural Selection of Populations and Communities.* Menlo Park, CA: Benjamin/Cummings.

Wilson, E.O. 1975. *Sociobiology: The New Synthesis.* Cambridge, MA: Harvard University Press.

————. 1978a. *On Human Nature.* Cambridge, MA: Harvard University Press.

————. 1978b. Academic vigilantism and the political significance of sociobiology. In *The Sociobiology Debate.* A.L. Caplan, editor. New York: Harper and Row.

Wilson, J.Q. and Herrnstein, R.J. 1985. *Crime and Human Nature.* New York: Simon and Schuster.

Wilson, M., Daly, M., and Weghorst, S.J. 1981. Differential maltreatment of girls and boys. *Victimology* 6:249.

Winnicott, D.W. 1958. *Collected Papers: Through Paediatrics to Psycho-Analysis.* New York: Basic Books.

Winokur, G. 1980. Is there a common genetic factor in bipolar and unipolar affective disorder? *Comprehensive Psychiatry* 21:460.

Winokur, G., Tsuang, M.T., and Crave, R.R. 1982. The Iowa 500: Affective disorder in relatives of manic and depressive patients. *American Journal of Psychiatry* 139:200.

Wolf, A.P. 1966. Childhood association, sexual attraction, and the incest taboo: A Chinese case. *American Anthropologist* 68:883.

————. 1968. Adopt a daughter-in-law, marry a sister: A Chinese solution to the problem of incest taboo. *American Anthropologist* 70:864.

————. 1970. Childhood association and sexual attraction: A further test of the Westermarck hypothesis. *American Anthropologist* 72:503.

Wolff, P.H. 1978. The biology of morals from a psychological perspective. In *Morality as a Biological Phenomenon*. G.S. Stent, editor. Berlin: Dahlem Konferenzen.

Wrangham, R.W. 1982. Mutualism, kinship and social evolution. In *Current Problems in Sociobiology*. King's College Sociobiology Group, editors. Cambridge: Cambridge University Press.

Wyer, R.S., and Srull, T.K., eds. 1984. *Handbook of Social Cognition*. Hillsdale, NJ: Lawrence Erlbaum.

———. 1986. Human cognition in its social context. *Psychological Review* 93:322.

Wynne, L.C., Toohey, M.L., and Doane, J. 1979. Family studies. In *Disorders of the Schizophrenic Syndrome*. L. Bellak, editor. New York: Basic Books.

Wynne-Edwards, V.C. 1962. *Animal Dispersion in Relation to Social Behaviour*. Edinburgh: Oliver and Boyd.

———. 1963. Intergroup selection in the evolution of social systems. *Nature* 200:623.

Yalom, I.D., Green, R., and Fisk, N. 1973. Prenatal exposure to female hormones. *Archives of General Psychiatry* 28:554.

Yamaguchi, M., Yanase, T. Nagamo, H., et al. 1970. Effect of inbreeding on mortality in Fukuoka population. *American Journal of Human Genetics* 22:145.

Yamaguchi, M., Yamazaki, K., Beauchamp, G.K., et al. 1981. Distinctive urinary odors governed by the major histo-compatibility locus of the mouse. *Proceedings of the National Academy of Science of the United States of America* 78:5817.

Young, L.D., Suomi, S.S., Harlow, H.F., et al. 1973. Early stress and later response to separation in rhesus monkeys. *American Journal of Psychiatry* 130:400.

Zeanah, C.H., and Zeanah, P.D. 1989. Intergenerational transmission of maltreatment: Insights from attachment theory and research. *Psychiatry* 52:177.

Ziegler, F.J., Imboden, J.B., and Meyer, E. 1960. Contemporary conversion symptomatology. *American Journal of Psychiatry* 116:901.

Zitrin, C.M., Klein, D.F., and Woerner, M.G. 1980. Treatment of agoraphobia with group exposure in vivo and imipramine. *Archives of General Psychiatry* 37:63.

———., et al. 1983. Treatment of phobias: I. Imipramine and placebo. *Archives of General Psychiatry* 40:125.

Zitrin, C.M., and Ross, D.C. 1988. Early separatio anxiety and adult agoraphobia. *Journal of Nervous and Mental Disease* 176:621.

Zivin, G., ed. 1985. *The Development of Expressive Behavior: Biology-Environment Interactions*. New York: Academic Press.

Zoccolillo, M., and Cloninger, C.R. 1986. Somatization disorder: Psychologic symptoms, social disability, and diagnosis. *Comprehensive Psychiatry* 27:65.

Index

About the Author

Brant Wenegrat is assistant professor of psychiatry and behavioral science at Stanford University School of Medicine, and chief of psychiatric clinical services at the Palo Alto Veterans' Administration Medical Center. He has lectured and written extensively about sociobiology and its relationship to psychiatry. He is the author of *Sociobiology and Mental Disorder* (1984) and *The Divine Archetype* (1990).